Developing the Digital Lung:
From First Lung CT to Clinical AI

The Development of Quantitative X-ray Computed
Tomography of Diffuse Lung Disease Through the
Use of Artificial Intelligence

Developing the Digital Lung: From First Lung CT to Clinical AI

The Development of Quantitative X-ray Computed Tomography of Diffuse Lung Disease Through the Use of Artificial Intelligence

JOHN D. NEWELL, Jr., MD, FACR

Elsevier
1600 John F. Kennedy Blvd.
Ste 1800
Philadelphia, PA 19103-2899

DEVELOPING THE DIGITAL LUNG   ISBN: 9780323795012

Notice

International Standard Book Number: 9780323795012

Content Strategist: Melanie Tucker
Content Development Specialist: Rebecca Corradetti
Publishing Services Manager: Shereen Jameel
Project Manager: Shereen Jameel
Design Direction: Margaret M. Reid

Printed in India

Last digit is the print number: 9 8 7 6 5 4 3 2 1

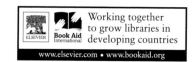

I dedicate this book to all who suffer from lung disease and to those who strive to research, diagnose, and treat lung disease.

ACKNOWLEDGMENTS

I want to express my deep thanks and gratitude to all my patients, mentors, students, and colleagues who have all taught me so much over the past 45 years. I want to thank all the people at Elsevier, and especially my editor, Rebecca Corradetti and Shereen Jameel, who helped me so much in improving the quality of this book.

I am a cardiothoracic radiologist and biomedical engineer with over 40 years of experience in clinical radiology, and teaching and research, most recently at the University of Iowa and VIDA. I have marveled for many years at the ability of x-ray computed tomography to generate 3D images of the lung for both visual interpretation and quantitative analysis. Computed tomography images of the lungs have been shown to be a powerful method of detecting and assessing a variety of lung diseases, including lung cancer, asthma, COPD, COVID-19, and pulmonary fibrosis. I was approached by Elsevier in December 2019 at the RSNA convention to write a book on medical imaging AI, and we agreed that a book on lung CT AI would be the best fit for both of us. I wrote this book between January 2020 and February 2021 in Port Townsend, Washington, where I live. I hope you enjoy reading the book as much as I did writing it.

CONTENTS

CHAPTER 1

Introduction to Lung CT AI

AI: An Intelligent Agent

The foundation for this book about lung CT AI is the application of what Alan Turing described in 1936 as the "universal Turing machine."[1] This is what is known today as the computer hardware and software that dominates so much of our lives, and is at the heart of lung CT AI. In his recent book, Stuart Russell describes succinctly what Alan Turing meant by the universal Turing machine.[1] The essence of Turing's discovery was to define two new mathematical objects. The first was defined as a machine, what is known today as computer hardware. The second, mathematical object, Turing defined as a program that is known as software code that runs on the computer hardware. Together, the machine (computer hardware) and the program (software code) define a sequence of events, or a sequence of state changes, that occur in the machine (computer CPU, computer memory, etc.) to accomplish a task.

Russell describes the key concept in modern artificial intelligence (AI) as being the concept of an intelligent agent.[1] The intelligent agent exists in the software programs running on a computer. How the AI agent is built depends on the objective(s) to be achieved or the problem(s) to be solved. The functioning AI agent then depends on four important things: (1) environment; (2) observations; (3) actions; and (4) objective(s)[1] (Fig. 1.1). The environment is the physical and electronic space that the AI agent can access. Using the word processing (WP) AI agent as an example, the WP AI agent environment includes keyboard commands, computer display, and computer hardware and software, as well as any internet connections that are running. The observations that the WP can make are the keystrokes pressed, and it can read the WP files that exist on the computer and in the cloud. The actions that the WP can take are: recording the keystrokes and displaying those on the screen; storing them on the computer or the Internet; and reading and writing existing WP files from the computer memory, hard disk drive, and the Internet (Fig. 1.2). The objectives for the WP AI agent are determined by the people who wrote the software to run on the computer. These objectives can be summarized as taking keystroke inputs and creating a software file that records the keystrokes and displays them on the computer screen. It is also important to recognize that one AI agent can pass the objectives to another AI agent to perform additional objectives, and this process can continue with as many AI agents as desired. For example, the WP files on a computer can be sent to a typesetting program that a publisher would use to generate the final output for a book.

AI DEFINITIONS AND LEVELS

AI is a rapidly expanding field, and definitions of the different levels of AI are changing as a result of this growth. AI, for the purpose of this book, includes four levels: (1)

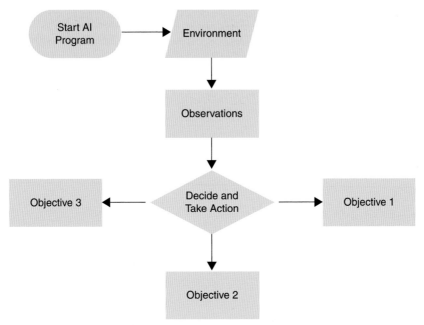

Fig. 1.1 The four elements of an intelligent agent (AI agent): environment, observations, actions, and objective(s).

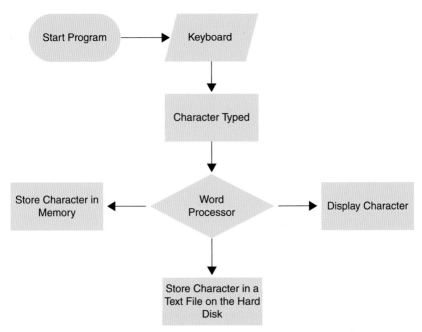

Fig. 1.2 How the four elements of an AI agent work to enable the objective(s) of a simple word processing program.

BOX 1.1 ■ Four Levels of Increasing AI Capabilities	
Level 1	Reactive Machine AI
Level 2	Limited-Memory AI
Level 3	Theory-of-Mind AI
Level 4	Self-Aware AI

reactive machine; (2) limited-memory; (3) theory of mind; and (4) self-aware[2] (Box 1.1). Since the late 1960s and early 1970s, reactive machine type AI has driven the development of multiple AI technologies to visually and, subsequently, quantitatively assess the presence and extent of lung diseases using x-ray CT scanning. More recently, limited-memory levels of AI have been added to the list of technologies driving progressive improvements in the visual and quantitative CT assessment of lung disease. Reactive machines are the most basic type of AI system. This means that they cannot form memories or use past experiences to influence presently made decisions; they can only react to currently existing situations—hence the term "reactive." An existing form of a reactive machine is Deep Blue, a chess-playing supercomputer created by IBM in the mid-1980s.[2] Reactive machine AI programs will only react in the present in the way they are programmed. Examples of reactive machine AI programs in CT lung AI would include analytic CT image reconstruction algorithms, analytic CT image lung segmentation programs, computing the lung CT image voxel histogram, and relevant voxel histogram statistics that have been previously shown to correlate with normal and diseased lung tissue. These reactive machine lung CT AI metrics of lung disease can be used to detect and assess the extent of normal and abnormal lung structure and function caused by underlying lung disease, such as emphysema, asthma, or pulmonary fibrosis. The advantage of reactive machine learning AI is that it is very clear what the software program is doing. However, it is not as powerful as limited-memory AI. Limited-memory AI is comprised of machine learning models that derive knowledge from previously learned information, stored data, or events. Unlike reactive machines, limited-memory learns from the past by observing actions, or data fed to them, in order to build experiential knowledge.[2] Limited-memory machine learning AI has been used in identifying specific patterns of lung disease, such as honeycombing in patients with ILD. Limited-memory machine learning AI has also been applied to CT image reconstruction, reducing noise in reconstructed CT images. It has also been implemented in segmentation software to extract the lungs from the rest of the thoracic anatomy on CT images. Limited-memory AI machine learning has been used to identify unique patient CT phenotypes in patients with COPD[3] and asthma.[4] Limited-memory AI machine learning has also been used to classify lung nodules into benign and malignant categories.[5]

Lung CT AI involves a number of simpler AI agents that are linked together to produce a final lung CT AI objective, which is to detect and assess normal and diseased lung structure and function and make these results widely available to patients and healthcare providers. The lung CT AI agents that are included in this book, in the order in which they are usually performed, are: (1) generate high-quality CT images of the thorax; (2) display the CT images of the thorax; (3) separate or segment the lung CT images from the rest of the thoracic anatomy; (4) extract quantitative features from the

lung CT images that represent meaningful metrics of normal and diseased lung structure and function; (5) analyze these features to predict the presence or absence of lung
disease, and to assess the extent and impact of any detected lung disease; and (6) make
these results available in near real time for patients and their health care providers (Fig.
1.3). The routine lung CT AI outputs for individual patient care can then be systemati-
cally collected and examined across healthcare systems and countries; these results can

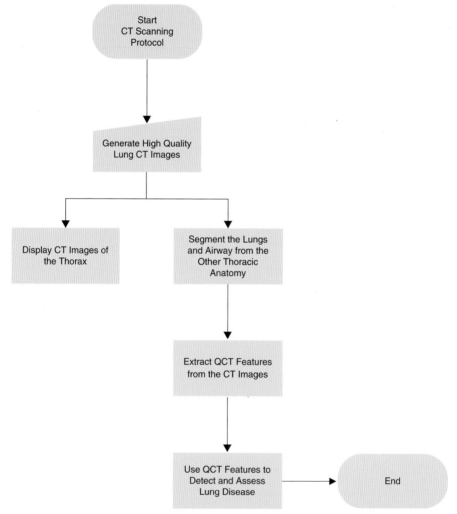

Fig. 1.3 The sequence of lung CT AI agents in the order in which they are performed: generate
high-quality CT images of the thorax, display the CT images of the thorax, separate or segment
the lung CT images from the rest of the thoracic anatomy, extract quantitative CT (QCT) features
from the lung CT images that represent meaningful metrics of normal and diseased lung structure
and function, analyze these features to predict the presence or absence of lung disease and to
assess the extent and impact of any detected lung disease, and make these results available in
near realtime for patients and their health care providers.

be used in near real time to assess world lung health and disease, and to inform how best to allocate scarce resources needed to decrease the prevalence and severity of lung disease. My biggest reason for writing this book is to make everyone aware that the lung CT AI objectives outlined above are now achievable. I believe lung CT AI will work best in a healthcare environment where everyone has access to quality healthcare, regardless of ability to pay or preexisting conditions.

This book will follow the sequence of AI agents that have been developed over the last 50 years to generate a 3D digital representation of the lung using x-ray CT,[6,7] and finally develop an AI agent that is useful in detecting and predicting the malignant potential of pulmonary nodules;[5] the presence and severity of diffuse lung diseases, such as chronic obstructive pulmonary disease (COPD),[8] idiopathic pulmonary fibrosis (IPF),[9] and, most recently, COVID-19 viral pneumonia.[10] The progressive improvements in CT scanner technology have advanced the 3D visualization of normal lung structure and function and made it possible to develop new AI methods to accurately detect and assess normal and diseased states of the lung. The progressive increases in our knowledge of lung CT AI will help guide our narrative from describing the first digital images of the lung obtained from x-ray computed tomography, to the very recent exciting application of quantitative CT AI methods for the detection and assessment of the severity of lung nodules and acute and chronic diffuse lung disease. The high spatial and contrast resolution of modern chest CT images of the lung has also enabled the creation of sophisticated software to build silicon computer models of normal and diseased lungs, and has increased our fundamental understanding of lung physiology and pathophysiology.[11,12]

Diagnosis of COPD, ILD, Lung Cancer, and Other Smoking-Related Diseases

The inhalation of cigarette smoke or other environmental combustion products is the leading cause of COPD and lung cancer. The inhalation of these combustion products leads to inflammation and oxidative stress in the lung tissues. COPD decreases the effectiveness of gas exchange through the destruction of alveolar walls and increases the resistance of getting gas to the alveoli through the narrowing and destruction of airways. The combination of these processes greatly impairs the function of the lungs in a COPD patient. COPD is the fourth leading cause of death in the United States behind heart disease, cancer, and accidental deaths.[13] COPD is usually diagnosed late in the course of the illness and is often misdiagnosed. Lung cancer screening in the United States, using low-dose chest CT scans, is an opportunity to detect early lung cancers caused by exposure to cigarette smoking, but also to diagnose COPD at earlier stages when there is more time to intervene and alter the course of the disease.

Earlier detection of chronic interstitial lung disease (ILD) provides the opportunity for early therapeutic intervention and improved patient outcomes.[14] Chronic ILD produced by IPF, HP, and CTD produces thickening of the alveolar walls, which decreases the efficiency of gas exchange. These diseases can also distort and destroy the normal architecture of the lung acinus, decreasing the effective surface–to–volume ratio of the lung. ILD is also a disease that is often diagnosed in more advanced stages and often misdiagnosed. People with IPF frequently have a significant history of cigarette smoking, and ILD is often present in patients with COPD.

Information for Healthcare Providers and Administrators, Patients, and Researchers

I believe there is a need for a book on lung CT AI to inform healthcare providers and administrators, patients, researchers, and government agencies about the development, validation, and commercial availability of lung CT AI products that can detect and assess several lung diseases, including lung cancer, COPD, COVID-19 pneumonia, and ILD. COPD and ILD are often diagnosed in later stages of the disease and often missed in the earlier stages of disease when the disease is more treatable. The lung CT AI assessment of COVID-19 viral pneumonia during the ongoing worldwide pandemic of 2020 has been helpful in countries and healthcare systems where access to timely quality RT-PCR testing is not available or is unreliable. Lung CT AI programs can help identify COVID-19 pneumonia from other forms of pneumonia and assess which patients will need to be hospitalized and are at increased risk of dying.

Lung cancer is the leading cause of cancer deaths in the United States, and there now exists AI software that can help identify benign versus malignant lung nodules.[5] Until recently, these lung CT AI technologies were only used in research studies because of the difficulty in deploying the software in busy radiology practices within clinics and hospitals. This has changed with the advent of software programs, like VIDA Insight, that can be deployed independently or in larger enterprise AI ecosystems of large computer companies.[15] Small agile software companies, like VIDA, can develop specialized AI software to assess lung CT images for the presence and severity of lung structural and functional changes due to disease, and these specialized AI software programs can now be accessed at the point of care without slowing down the radiology workflow; this novel CT lung AI software can increase efficiency in radiology practices. There are potential broader favorable impacts on human health than just the care of individual patients. QCT metrics of lung disease that are driven by environmental pollution, such as COPD and lung cancer, can be assessed in an objective way across hospital systems, states, and nations. This will inform governments and leaders on how best to spend limited resources on improving the environment and lessening the spread of environmentally driven lung diseases.

Describing Lung CT AI in Three Stages

This book includes a historical description of the technological developments that were necessary to achieve the current success of lung CT AI software in the clinical care of patients with lung disease. The structure of the book is divided into three segments. The first segment, Chapters 2 and 3, discusses the development of x-ray CT scanners and scanning protocols that are used to scan the thorax and generate 3D images of the lungs.

Chapter 2 begins with the invention of the x-ray computed tomographic (CT) scanner that, at first, could only generate a limited number of low-spatial-resolution contiguous 2D digital images of the thorax with a long scan time. The first whole-body CT scanner, ACTA CT scanner, had very slow scan times, 4.5 minutes to obtain two 7.5-mm nearly contiguous axial images of the thorax with a spatial resolution in the axial x-y plane of 1.5 mm and the z-axis of 7.5 mm.[6] The ACTA CT scan time for an adult male lung that is 30 cm in length would take a minimum of 90 minutes, longer if x-ray tube cooling was needed. The scan time and the spatial resolution of the CT scanner are important metrics that drive what can be done with AI in analyzing images of the lung. Chapter 2 also follows several key technologies that were developed to improve the spatial resolution and decrease scan times of x-ray CT scanners; scan time and spatial resolution have greatly improved over the last 40 years.

Chapter 3 discusses the latest generation of x-ray CT scanner technologies and lung CT scanning protocols available in 2020. The latest generation of CT scanners can scan the entire thorax in less than 10 seconds with an isotropic resolution of 0.5 mm. Chapter 3 details the important CT scanning variables that need to be carefully selected, such as x-ray dose, scan time, z-axis resolution, and image reconstruction method, to produce the best lung CT images.

The second segment of the book, Chapters 4 through 7, describes the lung CT AI methods that have been developed to detect and quantitatively assess focal lung nodules, pulmonary emphysema, pulmonary fibrosis, and acute COVID-19 viral pneumonia from the CT-generated density maps of the lung.

Chapter 4 discusses the concept of the lung nodule and how CT is used to detect and quantitatively assess the malignant potential of a lung nodule. Exposure to environmental factors, especially cigarette smoke, increases the risk of developing lung cancer. It has been shown recently that the use of screening lung CT scans can decrease mortality in people exposed to cigarette smoke.

Chapters 5, 6, and 7 introduce increasingly more sophisticated lung CT AI methods to assess diffuse lung disease, starting with CT image voxel histograms in Chapter 5 and ending with sophisticated limited-memory AI machine learning algorithms in Chapter 7.

Chapter 5 describes the QCT metrics that are readily obtained from a single total lung capacity (TLC) CT scan done with an appropriate CT protocol, as outlined in Chapter 3. Lung CT density metrics were the first lung CT AI metrics to be reported and focused mainly on the reduced density of the lung produced by pulmonary emphysema. Pulmonary fibrosis produces increased density in the lung and can also be assessed using density measures from lung CT images. Chapter 5 describes the research studies that were performed to determine if the QCT metrics described do, in fact, represent important features of normal and diseased lung tissue by correlating CT image findings to other measures of lung disease (e.g., pulmonary function tests, lung pathology). Chapter 5 discusses how quantitative CT lung images provide critical new information regarding COPD that was not obtained from other methods (e.g., clinical history, pulmonary function testing).[16] Determining the value of lung CT AI versus other means of assessing patients with COPD required the funding of large multicenter NIH grants that studied thousands of subjects with and without COPD. These studies established the relative value of lung CT AI metrics with other data characterizing COPD-related lung disease, including genetic studies, pulmonary physiology testing, and standardized healthcare questionnaires. These studies included COPDGene, MESA Lung, and SPIROMICS. One QCT lung AI study in the SPIROMCS study identified four unique clusters of subjects with COPD that had different QCT metrics and different disease trajectories.[3] Chapter 5 also discusses the results of multiple smaller-size research studies in assessing the value of lung CT AI in groups of patients with pulmonary fibrotic lung disease associated with idiopathic pulmonary fibrosis (IPF), connective tissue disease

(CTD), and hypersensitivity pneumonitis (HP). A number of QCT density metrics are shown to be effective in assessing pulmonary fibrosis in ILD. These metrics include whole lung histogram measurements of the lung and their associated statistics, including mean lung density, skewness, and kurtosis.[17,18] They also include QCT measures of the amount of lung density between -600 HU and -250 HU.[19]

Chapter 6 introduces dynamic QCT metrics that can be generated using two CT scans done sequentially at different lung volumes. These metrics provide a means of assessing lung structure and function. The assessment of lung ventilation can be done using an inspiratory and expiratory CT scan and looking at the change in lung density, or change in lung volume, between the two scans. There are several ways to apply this methodology to assessing lung ventilation at the whole lung level, lobe level, segment level, acinar level, and voxel level. Lung biomechanics can also be assessed using two chest CT scans obtained at different lung volumes, typically TLC and RV.

Chapter 7 looks at limited-memory type AI metrics in assessing COPD, ILD, and COVID-19 pneumonia. Limited-memory type AI algorithms are trained in three stages (Fig. 1.4) to detect and assess the presence of lung disease. The first stage is feature extraction. This can be done using supervised or unsupervised approaches. Supervised approaches have an expert imaging physician label the normal and abnormal tissue features on the lung CT images. Unsupervised approaches let the AI algorithm determine the normal and abnormal tissue types. The second stage used to train the AI algorithm is to have it recognize and quantitate the amount of the normal and abnormal tissue features, or textures, within the lung CT images that correspond to important pathologic features associated with different lung diseases. The number of supervised or unsupervised training CT cases can be increased to improve the performance of the limited-memory lung CT AI program. The design of the limited-memory lung CT AI program can also be altered to improve its performance. The third stage tests the performance of the trained AI algorithm on a test set of chest CT scans from a cohort of human subjects separate from the training cohort. The performance of the lung CT AI algorithm is based on its ability to identify the different tissue features on the test set of chest CT scans, including features such as emphysema, honeycombing, and consolidation.

The third segment of the book includes Chapters 8 and 9. Chapter 8 discusses the concept of physiomics. The goal of lung physiomics is to generate computer models of all the anatomical and physiologic functions of the lung to gain new insights into normal and diseased lung function. A specific lung physiome model of lung ventilation and perfusion are discussed that can be used to better assess the risk of acute pulmonary emboli (APE). APE can acutely increase the mean pulmonary artery pressure and induce right ventricular failure. Simply computing the volume of acute blood clots occluding the lumen of pulmonary arteries does not predict increased pulmonary artery pressures as accurately as the lung physiome model of ventilation and perfusion. 3D lung CT images provide the spatial information of lung structure for this lung physiome model. The lung physiome model builds a complete picture of lung structure and function across multiple spatial scales, physical functions, and their integration.

Chapter 9 discusses how the AI methods described in Chapters 2 through 8 can now be applied to the routine care of patients in the normal clinical workflow. This has been the goal of lung CT AI for many decades and is now possible in the 2020s due to numerous advances in computing that have occurred over the past three decades. One

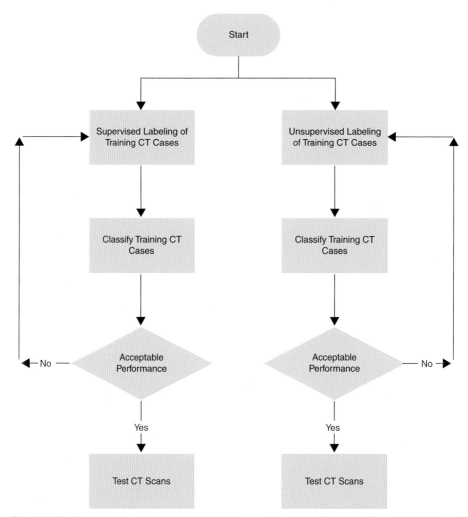

Fig. 1.4 The three steps used to train limited-memory type lung CT AI algorithms to detect and assess normal and diseased lung tissue. The first stage is feature extraction. This can be done using supervised or unsupervised approaches. Supervised approaches have an expert imaging physician label the normal and abnormal tissue features on the lung CT images. Unsupervised approaches let the AI algorithm determine by itself the normal and abnormal tissue types. The second stage trains the AI algorithm to recognize and quantitate the amount of the normal and abnormal tissue features, or textures, within the lung CT images that correspond to important pathologic features associated with different lung diseases. The number of supervised or unsupervised training CT cases can be increased to improve the performance of the limited-memory lung CT AI program. The design of the limited-memory lung CT AI program can also be altered to improve its performance. The third stage tests the performance of the trained AI algorithm on a test set of chest CT scans from a cohort of human subjects separate from the training cohort. The performance of the lung CT AI algorithm is based on its ability to identify the different tissue features on the test set of chest CT scans including features such as emphysema, honeycombing, and consolidation.

of the main goals of this book is to show how the advancement of lung CT AI over the past 45 years has made it possible to provide lung CT AI technologies in the current clinical medical imaging environment. These advances in computing have enabled the emergence of several small clinical CT lung AI imaging companies that began as research-only enterprises, to help provide the lung CT AI tools needed for large NIH studies such as COPDGene, Mesa Lung, and SPIROMICS. The success of lung CT AI in the research realm has motivated these small lung CT AI companies to develop new clinical products in lung CT AI.

VIDA is one of these companies that has developed lung CT AI software that can run independently, or on large enterprise-scale medical imaging AI ecosystems so that the previously validated quantitative CT metrics of lung disease can be extracted in near real time, and made available to the imaging and referring physician for the immediate care of the patient at the point of care. Chapter 9 reviews the current information technologies (IT) that are in use in modern healthcare hospitals and clinics to support the acquisition, storage, and distribution of medical imaging studies, including x-ray CT studies of the thorax and how the imaging IT interacts with the larger healthcare IT that supports the patient's electronic medical record (EMR). We then discuss the lung CT AI technology that is now available within the imaging IT ecosystem to automatically assess lung CT images for quantitative metrics of lung disease. Specifically, we discuss VIDA Insights v3.0 Density/tMPR module and Texture/Subpleural View module. Both use reactive machine AI and limited-memory AI methods to analyze each lung and lobe of a chest CT scan for the following quantitative CT metrics: lung and lobe volume in liters, LAA_{-950} metric for emphysema, $HAA_{-700\ to\ -250}$ metric for COVID-19 pneumonia and ILD, and the texture patterns that make up the $HAA_{-700\ to\ -250}$ that include ground-glass/reticular opacities, consolidation, and honeycombing. The chapter concludes by discussing the importance of responsible AI in any application of AI, along with guidelines to achieve responsible lung CT AI. The current technology state of lung CT AI can accomplish what could only have been dreamed about by investigators when the "Density Mask" CT technique was first published in 1988 as a CT method of assessing reduced lung density by emphysema.[20]

References

1. Russell S. *Human Compatable: Artificial Intelligence and the Problem of Control.* New York, NY: Viking; 2019:336.
2. Reynoso R. 4 Main Types of Artificial Intelligence. 2019. Available at: https://www.g2.com/articles/types-of-artificial-intelligence.
3. Haghighi B, Choi S, Choi J, Hoffman EA, Comellas AP, Newell Jr. JD, et al. Imaging-based clusters in current smokers of the COPD cohort associate with clinical characteristics: the SubPopulations and Intermediate Outcome Measures in COPD Study (SPIROMICS). *Respir Res.* 2018;19(1):178.
4. Choi S, Hoffman EA, Wenzel SE, Castro M, Fain S, Jarjour N, et al. Quantitative computed tomographic imaging-based clustering differentiates asthmatic subgroups with distinctive clinical phenotypes. *J Allergy Clin Immunol.* 2017;140(3):690–700.e8.
5. Uthoff J, Stephens MJ, Newell Jr. JD, Hoffman EA, Larson J, Koehn N, et al. Machine learning approach for distinguishing malignant and benign lung nodules utilizing standardized perinodular parenchymal features from CT. *Med Phys.* 2019;46(7):3207–3216.
6. Ledley RS, Di Chiro G, Luessenhop AJ, Twigg HL. Computerized transaxial x-ray tomography of the human body. *Science.* 1974;186(4160):207–212.

7. Schellinger D, Di Chiro G, Axelbaum SP, Twigg HL, Ledley RS. Early clinical experience with the ACTA scanner. *Radiology*. 1975;114(2):257–261.
8. Humphries SM, Notary AM, Centeno JP, Strand MJ, Crapo JD, Silverman EK, et al. Deep learning enables automatic classification of emphysema pattern at CT. *Radiology*. 2020;294(2):434–444.
9. Humphries SM, Yagihashi K, Huckleberry J, Rho BH, Schroeder JD, Strand M, et al. Idiopathic pulmonary fibrosis: data-driven textural analysis of extent of fibrosis at baseline and 15-month follow-up. *Radiology*. 2017;285(1):270–278.
10. Li L, Qin L, Xu Z, Yin Y, Wang X, Kong B, et al. Artificial intelligence distinguishes COVID-19 from community acquired pneumonia on chest CT. *Radiology*. 2020:200905.
11. Tawhai M, Clark A, Donovan G, Burrowes K. Computational modeling of airway and pulmonary vascular structure and function: development of a "lung physiome". *Crit Rev Biomed Eng*. 2011;39(4):319–336.
12. Tawhai MH, Bates JH. Multi-scale lung modeling. *J Appl Physiol. (1985)*. 2011;110(5):1466–1472.
13. Heron M. Deaths: leading causes for 2017. *National Vital Statistics Reports*. 2019;68(6):1–76.
14. Fischer A, Patel NM, Volkmann ER. Interstitial lung disease in systemic sclerosis: focus on early detection and intervention. *Open Access Rheumatol*. 2019;11:283–307.
15. VIDA. VIDA 2020. Available at: https://vidalung.ai.
16. Lowe KE, Regan EA, Anzueto A, Austin E, Austin JHM, Beaty TH, et al. COPDGene((R)) 2019: redefining the diagnosis of chronic obstructive pulmonary disease. *Chronic Obstr Pulm Dis*. 2019;6(5):384–399.
17. Best AC, Lynch AM, Bozic CM, Miller D, Grunwald GK, Lynch DA. Quantitative CT indexes in idiopathic pulmonary fibrosis: relationship with physiologic impairment. *Radiology*. 2003;228(2):407–414.
18. Best AC, Meng J, Lynch AM, Bozic CM, Miller D, Grunwald GK, et al. Idiopathic pulmonary fibrosis: physiologic tests, quantitative CT indexes, and CT visual scores as predictors of mortality. *Radiology*. 2008;246(3):935–940.
19. Podolanczuk AJ, Oelsner EC, Barr RG, Hoffman EA, Armstrong HF, Austin JH, et al. High attenuation areas on chest computed tomography in community-dwelling adults: the MESA study. *Eur Respir J*. 2016;48(5):1442–1452.
20. Muller NL, Staples CA, Miller RR, Abboud RT. "Density mask". An objective method to quantitate emphysema using computed tomography. *Chest*. 1988;94(4):782–787.

CHAPTER 2

Three-Dimensional (3D) Digital Images of the Lung Using X-ray Computed Tomography

This chapter will discuss the digital lung, x-rays, and key components of the x-ray CT scanner to help better understand lung CT AI scanning protocols, and to briefly review the historical progression of advancements in x-ray computed tomography of the lungs from the 1970s through the development of multidetector spiral CT (MDCT) scanners in the early 2000s. Each CT technology advancement improved visual and quantitative assessment of x-ray CT images of the lung. The challenges that needed to be overcome included decreasing the examination time, increasing the spatial resolution of the CT images, and decreasing the x-ray dose to the patient. Each of these improvements, during this timeframe, was very important toward enabling future AI approaches in the diagnosis and assessment of lung diseases.

The Digital Lung

The digital lung is defined as a true three-dimensional (3D) representation of the right and left lungs (Fig. 2.1A). The digital lung, using human whole-body x-ray CT scanners available in 2020, is a collection of volume elements (voxels) that collectively represent the lung, and each voxel is assigned a value that corresponds to the average linear attenuation of the x-ray photons by the lung tissue within that voxel (Fig. 2.1B). The average volume of both human lungs is about 5 liters.[1] The size of the voxel, using modern MDCT scanners, can be as small as 0.5 mm for each axis. The total number of voxels contained in the lungs, in this case, is 40 million voxels. The first in a series of lung CT AI agents is the computer program running the x-ray CT scanner. Its objective is to generate 3D digital images of the lung that can then be viewed by patients and their physicians. This digital lung is the environment that additional AI agents can observe and, depending on the actions available to the particular AI agent, achieve additional objectives, such as segmenting the lungs from the other thoracic tissue and analyzing the lung voxels for measures of normal and diseased lung tissue (see Chapters 4 through 7).

X-ray Computed Tomography

X-ray computed tomography is a transmission computed tomographic method through which a precisely collimated external x-ray beam is transmitted through the human thorax (Fig. 2.2); the location and energy intensity of the x-ray photons that are not scattered or absorbed by thoracic tissue are captured on an x-ray detector designed for this purpose.

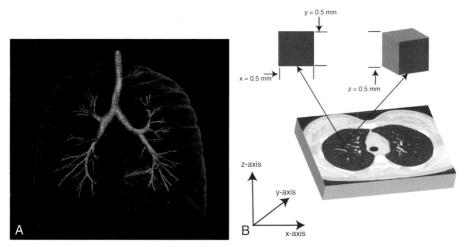

Fig. 2.1 **(A)** 3D rendering of both lungs obtained using a modern multidetector x-ray computed tomographic scanner and software to render the millions of voxels that were acquired into a single 3D rendering of the lungs. [Courtesy of VIDA.] **(B)** The cube shape of a 0.5-mm isotropic x-ray CT voxel is shown here and its relationship to a 2D axial chest CT image.

The x-ray CT scanner consists of several major components: x-ray tube and electronics, x-ray detector and electronics, CT gantry, patient table, computer hardware, software, and displays (Fig. 2.3). From the very first x-ray CT scanner to the current modern x-ray CT scanners of the 2020s, they all have needed these components to produce and display a CT image.[2] The advances in CT technology over the past five decades were made possible by advances in each of these key x-ray CT scanner components. It should be emphasized that without the AI software program running the x-ray CT scanner, there would be no practical way to reconstruct the CT images. The advent of relatively small and capable minicomputers in the 1960s made it possible to construct commercially viable x-ray CT scanners. The basic design of CT scans from the 1970s to the present share several common design features. Since the advent of human CT scans, it has been desirable to have the patient lay still in a supine position on the CT "scanning" table. The table moves the patient along their long axis, head-to-toe or z-axis, so the entire body can be scanned, if desired. The need to obtain multiple 1D projections of the supine patient laying in one position on the scanning table led to a CT scanner design where the x-ray tube rotates around the supine stationary subject with its corresponding x-ray detector on the opposite side of the patient (Fig. 2.4). The x-ray tube produces a beam of x-rays and these x-ray beams can have several geometric shapes including pencil beam, broad parallel beam, fan beam, or cone beam, depending on the CT scanner design. The most common current configuration of the x-ray beam is a rotating 50- to 60-degree cone beam (Fig. 2.5). The shape of the x-ray beam determines the shape of the x-ray detector array. The rotation axis of the x-ray tube and x-ray detector assembly is around the z-axis of the subject, and the highly collimated x-ray beam travels through the patient and onto the x-ray detectors. Today, the xy and z-axis width of individual detectors is less than 1 mm depending on the x-ray CT scanner model.

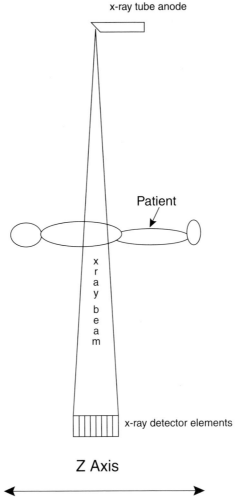

Fig. 2.2 Graphical representation of a tightly collimated x-ray beam in the z-axis that is transmitted through the thorax of a subject. The tightly collimated x-ray beam reduces the ionizing radiation exposure to adjacent tissues and increases the contrast resolution of the scan over what is possible with projection radiography, also shown here.

There are other medical imaging techniques that can generate 3D digital images of the lung; including magnetic resonance computed tomography (MRI), single-photon emission computed tomography (SPECT), positron emission computed tomography (PET), and hybrid imaging that combines two of these techniques (e.g., PET/CT, SPECT/CT, PET/MRI). X-ray transmission computed tomography (CT) is the most widely available computed tomographic method and is uniquely capable of rapid 3D imaging of the lungs, with both high image contrast and high spatial resolution, linear density scale over typical lung density values (−1000 HU to 0 HU), low claustrophobia, and low dose radiation (0.15 mGy to 1.5 mGy using modern x-ray CT scanners).[3]

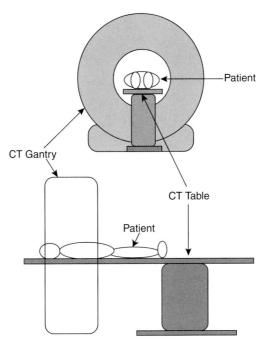

Fig. 2.3 Several major components of an x-ray CT scanner, including the gantry containing the x-ray tube, high energy voltage generator and corresponding x-ray detectors, and the CT scanning table with a patient positioned supine at the isocenter of the gantry. The CT technologist's computer and monitors are typically located in an adjoining room.

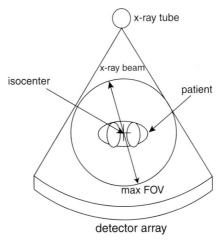

Fig. 2.4 The geometric relationships of the x-ray tube, patient, maximum scan field of view, and the x-ray detector array of third-generation CT scanner. Many 1D projections of the patient's anatomy are obtained as the x-ray tube and x-ray detector move around the patient on the CT scanning table. The patient is positioned at the isocenter of rotation of the CT gantry. The maximum scan field of view is indicated. The reconstruction or display field of view (DFOV) can be smaller than the maximum scan field of view.

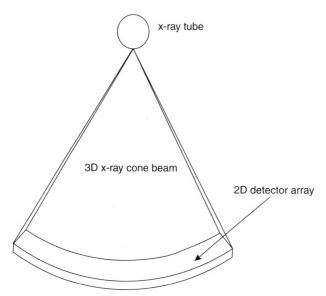

Fig. 2.5 Narrow 3D cone x-ray cone beam and its corresponding curved 2D x-ray detector array. This is the most common current geometric configuration of the x-ray beam and detector array used in clinical x-ray CT scanners.

The arrival of MDCT scanners in the 2000s, with 64 or more z-axis detector channels, has fueled multiple high-quality research studies that have increased our understanding of lung CT AI, its application in detecting, and assessing lung cancer and diffuse lung disease. Many research studies that have been done using x-ray CT in assessing COPD, ILD, and lung cancer, and these research studies provide the scientific foundations for this book (see Chapters 4 through 8).

X-RAYS

There are two forms of ionizing electromagnetic radiation, x-rays, and gamma rays. They are both high-energy photons capable of breaking covalent chemical bonds and because they can break covalent chemical bonds, are referred to as ionizing electromagnetic radiation.[4] Liquid water is the most abundant molecule in the human body and the ionization energy to remove an electron from water is 11.2 electron volts (eV).[4] A photon with an energy equal to or greater than 11.2 eV is considered ionizing radiation.[4] Covalent organic chemical bonds link together atoms in carbon-based living organisms and breaking these bonds can have serious consequences for the organism. The 3D distribution of energy concentration in units of joules per kilogram of the x-ray photons passing through the body is referred to as ionizing radiation absorbed dose. X-ray and gamma-ray photons are defined by how they are produced. The x-ray is produced outside the nucleus of an atom. In contrast, gamma rays are produced within the nucleus of the atom through radioactive decay of an excited nucleus. The energy of the gamma-ray is equal to the difference in the initial excited energy state of the nucleus and a lower state, or a ground state, of the nucleus.

The differential attenuation of the x-ray beam photons in biologic material provides the mechanism to generate diagnostic medical images of the human body. The differential attenuation of the photons involves elastic (Rayleigh) scattering of x-ray photons, photoelectric absorption of x-ray photons, and Compton scattering of x-ray photons, as the principal mechanisms of differential attenuation of the x-ray beam (using peak x-ray tube voltages (kVp) between 25 kV and 150 kV).[5] The dominant attenuation mechanism of x-rays in lung tissue and other soft tissue using a kVp between 70 kV and 150 kV (typical of non-contrast x-ray CT of the thorax) is Compton scattering.[5] The probability of a Compton scattering event per unit mass of incident x-rays on low atomic number materials (typical of normal lung tissue) is nearly independent of the atomic number (Z) of the scattering lung tissue.[5] The probability of a Compton scattering event per unit volume of incident x-rays on low atomic number materials is proportional to the density of the material.[5] The reason for this is, except for the hydrogen atom, the number of electrons per gram of tissue for low atomic number materials, such as carbon and oxygen, is relatively constant, so the number of electrons per gram of tissue is driven mainly by tissue density; the result is that the attenuation of x-rays in the lung tissue is proportional to the density of the lung tissue.[5] A good friend and colleague of mine, Jim Hogg, MD, has likened the x-ray CT scanner to a lung densitometer, and the above discussion supports this view. Photoelectric absorption of x-rays does come into play when intravenous iodinated contrast material is given to the patient just before the scan is performed. The presence of a high-atomic-number material like iodine (Z = 53, with a K shell orbital electron binding energy of 33 kV) will mean that the absorption of incident x-rays by iodine atoms will depend primarily on the photoelectric effect when incident x-rays interact with an iodine atom.[5]

IMPORTANT COMPONENTS OF AN X-RAY COMPUTED TOMOGRAPHIC (CT) SCANNER

CT X-ray Tube

The production of x-rays for medical imaging purposes is achieved by using an x-ray tube. The x-ray tube is a vacuum tube that has a very low internal pressure so that the interior of the x-ray tube contains very few atoms that would otherwise attenuate the flow of electrons in the x-ray tube. The x-ray tube contains a cathode, typically a coiled tungsten wire, at one end of the tube and an anode, typically a flat tungsten target, at the other end of the x-ray tube.[6] A current is passed through the cathode tungsten wire, which heats the wire, and the thermionic emission of electrons results in free electrons coming from the cathode.[6] The electrons are accelerated from the negatively charged cathode to the positively charged anode by placing a high voltage between the cathode and the anode. This voltage ranges from 25 kV to 150 kV in medical imaging. When the high-energy free electrons collide with an anode, made of a suitable material, x-ray photons are produced. Tungsten (W, Z = 74) is one of five refractory metals in the periodic table (Nb, Mo, Ta, W, Re) and has the second-highest atomic number (Z = 74) of the refractory metals. The higher the atomic number, the greater the production of x-rays with energies that are high enough for use in x-ray CT of the lung. Tungsten has the highest melting point and lowest vapor pressure of all metals, and at temperatures over 1650°C has the highest tensile strength.[7] Tungsten is a refractory metal with very high resistance to heat and wear, as well as a high atomic number (Z = 74), so it is an ideal anode target material. A Tungsten (90%)-Rhenium (Re, Z = 75) (10%) alloy can be used to increase the resistance to anode surface damage.[6]

The impact of the electrons on a tungsten metal anode produces the x-ray photons using two different methods: characteristic x-ray photon method and Bremsstrahlung x-ray photon method.[6] The characteristic x-rays are generated when an electron with sufficient kinetic energy strikes and ejects an inner electron (K electron orbit) in material with a high atomic number (Z), such as tungsten (W, Z = 74). Subsequently, an outer electron with the same high Z material transitions to the vacancy in the inner electron orbital and, in this process, an x-ray photon is generated with energy equal to the difference in the binding energy of the outer electron and the inner electron that was ejected. X-ray photons greater than 100 eV are termed characteristic photons whose energies are determined by the metal anode target. The most energetic characteristic x-rays from tungsten are due to transitions from the L (57.98 keV, 59.32 keV), or M shell (67.24 keV) to the K shell of tungsten.[6] The Bremsstrahlung, or breaking method of x-ray production, involves the deceleration of electrons as they penetrate a high Z anode target material, such as tungsten, and the deceleration of the electrons generates x-rays with photon energies between the working function of the metal and the keV used in the x-ray tube. The Bremsstrahlung x-rays are usually more abundant than characteristic x-rays in a CT scanner x-ray tube. The efficiency of generating Bremsstrahlung x-rays increases with the atomic number of the anode (Z = 74 for tungsten) and with the kilovoltage that is applied between the cathode and the anode.[6]

Modern x-ray tubes designed to be used with x-ray CT scanners have high power ratings, 5–7 megajoules, to be able to produce a large number of x-ray photons in a very short period of time.[1] The size of the x-ray tube focal spot on the tungsten anode is an important factor in determining the spatial resolution of the CT scanner. A smaller focal size can improve spatial resolution. However, a smaller focal spot size decreases the maximum number of x-ray photons that can be produced in a given period of time. Selection of the optimum focal spot size is an important CT scanning protocol variable for lung CT AI. The focal spot size of current x-ray CT scanners ranges from 1 to 2 mm.[1]

The x-ray tube peak kilovoltage (kVp) and tube current (mA) are two key variables in a lung CT scanning protocol. The kVp determines the x-ray beam peak energy, x-ray beam energy spectrum, and the efficiency of producing x-rays. The increase in efficiency of photon production will increase the ionizing radiation dose to the patient. The higher the kVp, the greater efficiency of producing x-rays for a given tube current. The higher the kVp (between 70 kV and 150 kV), the lower the tissue contrast. It is important in quantitative CT work to agree on the same kVp, since different kVp settings will change the HU values assigned to lung voxels for a given mA. The higher the kVp, the more efficient the x-ray photon production, so for a given mA, a higher kVp will result in higher radiation absorbed dose to the patient. For a given kVp, the tube current will determine the amount of x-ray photons produced. The higher the tube current, the more x-ray photons are produced for a given kVp. A higher tube current results in less image noise, but also higher radiation absorbed dose to the patient for a given kVp.

The x-ray tube current in mA determines the number of electrons that are accelerated between the x-ray tube cathode and anode per unit time. The tube current in mA multiplied by the length of time the x-ray tube is turned on, exposure time in seconds is called the tube current-time product or mAs. The mAs is proportional to the total number of x-ray photons the x-ray tube produces. The higher the mAs, the greater the number of x-ray photons produced and the higher ionizing radiation absorbed dose to the patient. The selection of a mAs value has a direct effect on the image noise and the radiation dose to the patient. Lung CT scanning protocols use mAs values that ensure adequate image quality with the lowest amount of radiation dose to the patient or subject being scanned.

Modern x-ray CT scanners use a bow tie-shaped x-ray beam filter to shape the beam so that all the detector elements in the detector array see a more uniform number of photons per unit area striking them.[1] The use of additional x-ray beam filtration can also modify the spectrum and intensity of the x-ray beam before it is transmitted through the patient. The addition of 5–10 mm thick aluminum filters in x-ray CT imaging will decrease the amount of lower energy x-rays that cannot penetrate the thickness of the thorax and contribute to the formation of the image, and also increase the fraction of higher energy photons that can reach the x-ray detector if they are not scattered or absorbed.[1]

It is now possible to control the kVp and mAs on modern CT scanners in realtime, and these values can be adjusted to provide a consistent signal-to-noise ratio in the CT image and a lower and more uniform radiation dose to the imaged tissues. These are referred to as tube kilovoltage modulation and tube current modulation (Fig. 2.6). The use of mA modulation in lung CT AI work has been successfully implemented recently. The use of kVp modulation is an issue in lung CT AI work when CT image voxel density values need to be consistent across time and patients. The varying kVp will change the x-ray beam energy spectrum, hence the CT image contrast and voxel density values will vary in the lung in a way that is challenging to correct at the present time.

In summary, the important factors regarding the operation of the x-ray tube that need to be factored into a CT scanning protocol include focal spot size, tube current-time product (mAs), peak kilovoltage (kVp), additional x-ray beam filtration, tube current modulation, and kilovoltage modulation.

CT X-ray Beam Shape and Energy Spectrum

The x-ray photon beam has several properties that impact scan time, image contrast, and ionizing radiation dose. Beam intensity and cross-sectional size of the photon beam determine how much tissue can be imaged per unit time. For a given beam intensity, the larger the cross-sectional size of the beam, the shorter time it takes to scan the lungs. The early CT scanners had very narrow pencil or rod-shaped photon beam cross-sections. This limitation was due to the reconstruction algorithms that were used, as well as limitations in the x-ray tube power and available x-ray detectors. The scan times were very long. The size of the x-ray beam cross-section has steadily increased over time as corresponding increases in x-ray tube output, x-ray detector array size, and computer power have been able to deal with large amounts of data per unit time coming from the x-ray detectors.

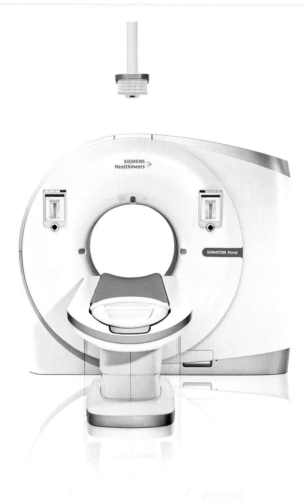

Fig. 2.6 Modern x-ray dual source multidetector CT scanner, Siemens SOMATOM FORCE CT scanner, showing the patient table in relationship to the large aperture of the CT gantry. *Courtesy Siemens Healthineers.*

The x-ray beam photon energy spectrum that irradiates the patient is a major factor in the image contrast of the final CT image. This energy spectrum needs to be carefully selected so that adequate image signal to noise ratio and contrast to noise ratio are present in the lung CT images at the lowest possible radiation dose. The energy spectrum needs to be the same in order to compare one patient to another and to assess the same patient at multiple time points. This is an important concept in quantitative CT of the lung because the values of the linear absorption coefficients, which determine the value assigned to each voxel in the image, are a function of the x-ray beam energy spectrum. To be able to compare voxel values over time from the same lung, or between lungs of different individuals, the x-ray energy spectrum needs to be the same. The photon energy spectrum for x-ray CT scanners is determined by the peak kilovoltage applied across the x-ray tube cathode and anode, and the type and thickness of metal filters placed in the path of the x-rays emitted from the x-ray tube anode. Higher x-ray tube peak kilovoltage (kVp) will shift the peak energy and the entire energy spectrum toward higher energies, and also increase the number of x-ray photons generated for a given mA setting. Lower peak kilovoltage will shift the peak energy and the energy spectrum to lower energies and decrease the number of photons generated for a given mA setting. The addition of metal filters between the x-ray tube anode and the patient can further shape the energy spectrum without increasing the peak energy by filtering out lower energies that are not able to penetrate the patient and reach the x-ray detectors. The peak kilovoltage and metal filters need to be carefully selected to optimize image quality and minimize the radiation dose to the patient or subject.

X-ray CT Detectors

The x-ray CT photon detectors that have been used since the first commercial CT scanners made in the 1970s to the current generation of CT scanners use energy integrating detectors (EID). The total energy of one or more photons that a single EID detector element measures during the measurement time are integrated to provide a total energy signal. This signal is often produced by many different photons of different energies. There are new commercial CT scanners in development that use photon-counting detectors (PCD). The photon-counting CT scanners detect each photon and its energy. The PCD CT scanners compared to the current EID CT scanners have the potential to further reduce radiation dose, increase image contrast and spatial resolution, correct beam hardening artifacts, improve CT intravenous contrast media enhanced imaging, and create new quantitative metrics for lung CT AI.[8]

The x-ray CT detectors are located opposite the x-ray tube. The x-ray CT detectors detect photons that are not scattered or absorbed by the tissues. These photons are transmitted through the tissue, without being scattered or absorbed, and then are detected by the x-ray detectors. The different tissues scatter/absorb the x-ray photons differently, so the number of and energy of x-ray photons that impact the x-ray detectors is related to the thickness and specific composition of the tissues imaged. The EID type detector elements are typically made from high-density ceramics containing rare earth materials, for instance, gadolinium oxysulfide (Gd_2O_2S).[1] The ceramic material is at the front of the individual detector element and absorbs the transmitted x-ray photons coming from the patient. Visible light is emitted by the ceramic material. This light is detected by an array of electronic solid-state photodiodes that register the location and total energy of the absorbed photons during a very short measurement time interval.[1] The electronic signal from the photodiodes is then digitized by an analog to digital converter and these digital signals are sent to the CT scanner's computer.

The physical size and shape of the detector array are determined by the shape of the x-ray beam. The current x-ray CT scanners use a narrow-angle cone beam, so the x-ray detector is a two-dimensional curved surface. The detector curvature is optimized to minimize differences in path length from the x-ray source to a given detector element. The size of the individual x-ray detector elements determines the maximum spatial resolution possible for the CT scanner. The rotation speed of the CT x-ray tube detector pair determines how fast the thorax can be scanned; all other factors held constant. The current generation of commercial CT scanners have a 360-degree rotation time as short as 0.25 seconds.

CT Gantry

The CT gantry has a large aperture at its center for the patient and the patient table to transit (Fig. 2.6). The modern CT gantry consists of two concentric cylinders, slip ring design, where the x-ray tube, x-ray detectors, and electronics, including the high voltage generator, rotate around the patient continuously. The control signals and scan data are transmitted from the rotating cylinder to the outer stationary cylinder (Fig. 2.7). The x-ray tube and corresponding detector array maintain an accurate fixed alignment with each other as they rotate around the patient. The x-ray photons that pass through the object are detected by the corresponding detector array located opposite the x-ray tube that is aligned with the detector array. Most CT scanners have a single x-ray tube and corresponding x-ray detector, but Siemens has made dual source CT scanners for over 15 years, which have two x-ray tubes and two corresponding x-ray detectors 90 degrees apart (Fig. 2.8). The current third-generation dual-source CT scanners have effective scan times that are half the scan times of similar single-source CT scanners. The dual-source CT scanner enables dual-energy CT imaging as well.

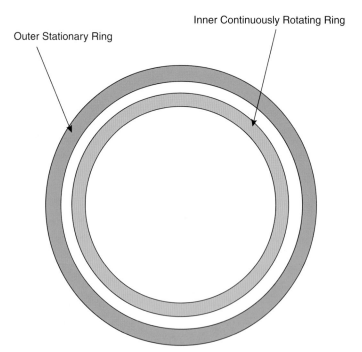

Fig. 2.7   Diagram of the concentric cylinder, or slip ring arrangement, of a spiral CT scanner. The inner ring rotates continuously around the patient while the outer ring is stationary.

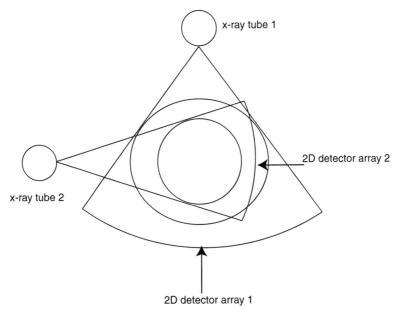

Fig. 2.8 Multidetector dual source CT (MDCT) scanners have two x-ray tubes and corresponding x-ray detector arrays that both rotate continuously around the patient. There is a 90-degree offset between the two x-ray tubes. When both x-ray systems are collecting data, the data collection rate is doubled for each 180 degrees of rotation. This enables very short scan times that are critical in cardiac CT imaging and combined cardiac and lung CT imaging. The maximum scan field of view of x-ray tube 1 is typically greater than the maximum scan field of view of x-ray tube 2 due to the constraints on space. The maximum field of view for dual acquisitions is limited to the maximum field of view of x-ray tube 2. Dual acquisitions can be used to increase data collection rates by a factor of two or to obtain acquisitions at two different x-ray tube kVps to generate dual energy CT scans.

CT Table, Isocenter, Scan Pitch, and Scanning Modes

The CT table in modern x-ray CT scanners is computer controlled and can position the patient very precisely on the x, y, and z-axis. Isocenter is an important CT scanning protocol parameter and refers to positioning the patient at the geometric center of the CT gantry aperture. The table can be lowered for ease of getting the patient on and off, and the table can be raised to precisely position the patient so that the center mass of the patient's thorax is at the isocenter of the CT gantry aperture. It is very important to scan the patient at the isocenter for visual or quantitative CT applications.[9–11] During spiral CT scanning, the CT table needs to accurately and precisely position the patient in response to commands from the CT scanner. This includes accurate and precise positioning of the patient while the table moves at relatively high speeds in the z-axis direction. The combination of the continuously rotating x-ray tube, x-ray detector within the CT gantry, and the moving CT table enables spiral CT scanning modes where the patient is moved continuously through the CT gantry, and a spiral path is traced out by the x-ray tube and x-ray detector relative to the patient. The tightness of this spiral path is the scan pitch. Pitch is an important CT protocol metric that needs to be set in the CT scanning protocol. Pitch is defined as the table feed distance per 360-degree rotation of the x-ray tube and x-ray detector array divided by the z-axis width of the x-ray detector array.

$$\text{Pitch} = (\text{Table Feed Distance per 360-degree rotation})/$$
$$(\text{z-axis width of the x-ray detector array})$$

A table speed of 80 mm/second, 360-degree gantry rotation time of 0.5 seconds, and a z-axis detector array width of 40 mm would result in a spiral CT scanning pitch of 1.0. A pitch of 1.0 in spiral CT scanning mode generates CT images that are similar to contiguous axial scanning mode (see Scanning Modes). The radiation dose is inversely proportional to the pitch. Pitch values higher than 1.5 enable faster scanning, lower radiation dose, and lower image quality. Pitch values less than 1.5 results in slower scanning, higher radiation dose, and higher image quality (Fig. 2.9). The pitch value usually chosen for lung CT AI are 1.0 or very close to it.

Scanning Modes

The two CT scanning modes available for lung CT are spiral mode and axial mode. Spiral mode is the main mode that that is currently used in lung CT AI protocols. Spiral mode involves moving the CT table that the patient rests on through the CT gantry aperture as the x-ray tube and x-ray detector array rotate continuously around the patient, see Fig. 2.9. Axial CT scanning mode keeps the patient table stationary as the x-ray tube and x-ray detector array rotate around the patient and, after a 360-degree rotation, the CT table moves the z-axis length of the x-ray detectors, and another set of axial mode CT images are obtained. Axial CT scanning mode was the first CT scanning mode that began in 1972 with the first EMI head CT scanner.

X-ray CT Scanning Modes

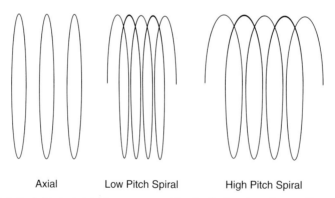

Axial   Low Pitch Spiral   High Pitch Spiral

Fig. 2.9 The x-ray tube and detector array, combined with the changing position of the patient being scanned as the CT table moves, trace out at a circle in axial scanning mode and a spiral/helical path in spiral scanning mode. This figure shows axial, low-pitch spiral and high-pitch spiral x-ray CT scanning modes. The low-pitch spiral has the spiral loops closely spaced, while the high-pitch spiral has the loops widely spaced. The pitch setting for lung CT AI work is typically 1 or close to 1.

Spiral CT scanning began in the late 1980s and early 1990s. Both spiral and axial CT scanning modes are used today depending on the CT scanner being used and the body part being scanned.

Collection of a Scanned Object's Projection Data

The primary objective of the CT AI agent that controls the actual scanning is to collect 1D projections from the x-ray detector array. The precise and accurate production of these 1D projections is very important in both visual and quantitative lung CT AI.

Image Reconstruction

The 1D projections that the CT scanner generates are considered forward projections of the object being scanned. These projections are log-transformed since the x-ray attenuation process is an exponential one, and the log transformation makes the reconstruction process a linear problem rather than an exponential problem.[1] The linear problem is easier to solve. The computer can reconstruct the object by back projection of the log-transformed projections to reconstruct the object of interest (Fig. 2.10). This back projection process is an inverse problem that attempts to reconstruct a 2D object from a set of 1D projections that are obtained at different angles of the x-ray tube and detector array. Simple back projection will cause blurring of the original object, (Fig. 2.10). The blurring can be corrected by using a deconvolution kernel.[1] This deconvolution kernel

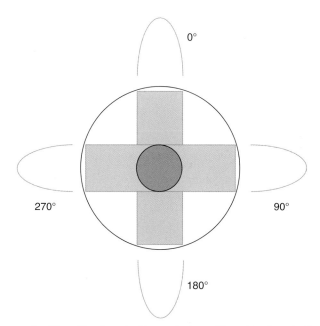

Fig. 2.10 Process of unfiltered back projection and why unfiltered back projection needs a correction factor or filter to create an accurate 2D image of an object from a set of 1D projections. The is an example of four 1D projections of a 2D circular object that are back projected and form a 2D star pattern, not the original 2D circular object.

is designed to undo the blurring caused by simple back projection. The deconvolution kernel is combined with each projection in a mathematical process called convolution. The original projections are each corrected by this convolution process. This process of correcting the blurring in the projections, and then back projection of the corrected or deblurred projections, is referred to as filtered back projection (FBP) (Fig. 2.10). It should be noted that inverse Radon transforms, as well as Fourier transforms, can be used in both unfiltered and FBP image reconstruction to recover a 2D image from a set of 1D projections of the object.[1] There are several available deconvolution kernels for x-ray CT scanners, and they have a big impact on the value of the CT numbers assigned to each image voxel. These CT numbers are the cornerstone of all AI applications involving x-ray CT of the lungs. Careful selection of the reconstruction method and reconstruction kernel in the CT scanning protocol is very important to achieve optimal results in lung CT AI.

FBP Versus Iterative Reconstruction Methods. The weighted FBP reconstruction method is an efficient analytical method to reconstruct images from a set of 1D projections of an object. The selection of specific reconstruction kernels will result in images with well-known noise structure and texture.[12] It is computationally very efficient and was, until recently, the most common mode of reconstruction for lung CT AI work. FBP is a linear method, so image quality can be assessed with a number of well-understood methods including standard deviation (SD) of CT numbers in a defined region of interest, signal-to-noise ratio (SNR), contrast-to-noise ratio (CNR), point and line spread functions to assess spatial resolution, modulation transfer function (MTF) to assess spatial resolution as a function of image contrast, and noise power spectrum (NPS).[12] The implementation of the FBP reconstruction method has been similar across multiple CT scanner manufacturers and x-ray CT scanner models. The main difference in the FBP method across different x-ray CT scanner models have been the deconvolutional kernel that is used to deblur the reconstructed images. By specifying a comparable kernel for each CT scanner model used in a CT scanning protocol, the values of the CT numbers obtained across different CT models and manufacturers can be standardized.

Until recently, the computational resources to implement iterative reconstruction methods of the 1D projection data for x-ray CT were too demanding. This has now changed with the increased computer power available in the 2020 s. The latest version of iterative reconstruction is described as model-based iterative reconstruction (MBIR).[12] MBIR begins with back projecting the measured projection data using the first iteration of the reconstructed image. Then a model of the CT imaging process is applied to the first iteration of the reconstructed image and this image undergoes forward projection to become a new updated projection of the measured projection data. This is repeated for all projections and then these are back projected to arrive at an updated and improved reconstructed image. This process is repeated until the improvement in the image reaches a plateau or some predetermined metric.[12] The advantages of the MBIR process include decreasing the image noise for a given x-ray dose or lowering the dose to obtain the same image noise, but with a lower radiation dose. The model of the CT imaging process can include CT system statistics and optics.[12] CT system statistics can include the x-ray tube photon beam spectrum, statistical distribution of the photon beam energies, and noise characteristics of the x-ray detectors and electronics. The

CT system optics include information about the geometry of the CT system. This can include the distance between the x-ray tube and the gantry isocenter, distance between the x-ray tube and the detectors, x-ray tube focal spot size and shape, size and shape of the individual detector elements, and the size and shape of the x-ray beam and detector array.[12] The more detailed the MBIR model of the CT imaging process, the greater the demands will be on computational resources. There is a tradeoff in the robustness of the MBIR model of the CT imaging process and the reconstruction times needed in a busy clinical practice.

The reduction in image noise for a given radiation dose is the compelling advantage of IR versus FBP methods of image reconstruction. The main disadvantage of IR is that it is a non-linear image reconstruction method, so the use of image quality metrics, such as SNR, CNR, MTF, and NPS, assume a linear and stationary imaging system. It is important in lung CT AI to assess image quality objectively. Improved methods to accurately assess MBIR CT images are needed.[12]

Scan Field of View (SFOV), Display Field of View (DFOV), and Reconstruction Matrix Size

Several other important parameters need to be optimized for lung CT AI work. These include scan field of view (SFOV), display field of view (DFOV), and the reconstruction matrix that is superimposed on the DFOV. The SFOV is the x–y-plane area that is scanned and is greater than or equal to the DFOV (Fig. 2.11). The DFOV is the actual x–y-plane area that is used to reconstruct a CT image (Fig. 2.11). The DFOV can be

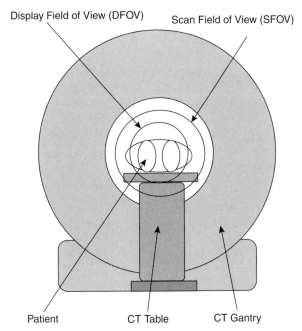

Fig. 2.11 CT gantry and table with the SFOV and corresponding DFOV relative to the position of the patient.

less than or equal to the SFOV. You might wonder, why bother with the DFOV? The additional parameter that needs to be considered is the size of the reconstruction voxel matrix that is superimposed on the DFOV. The current reconstruction matrix size is 512 × 512, but 1024 × 1024 is available for some CT scanner models. The size of the reconstruction matrix has a big impact on the speed at which images can be reconstructed and the size of these images. The larger the matrix, the greater the computing and storage resources necessary to reconstruct, display, and store the images. However, the larger the matrix size, the smaller the voxel size; hence, the greater the in plane or x–y-plane resolution. For a given x-ray dose, the smaller the voxel size, the greater the image noise. For example, if you doubled the matrix size, you would need to increase the x-ray dose by a factor of four to achieve the same signal-to-noise ratio for the measured Hounsfield number assigned to each of the smaller voxels in the reconstructed image. The x–y-plane dimensions of the reconstructed voxel for a 512 × 512 reconstruction matrix are driven by the following relationship:

$$X - Y = DFOV/512$$

For example, if the DFOV is 350 mm, the x–y dimensions of the reconstructed voxel would be 0.68 mm. If the DFOV is 500 mm, the x–y dimensions of the reconstructed voxel would be 0.98. This is a 50% increase in the x–y dimensions of the reconstructed voxel. For these reasons, the DFOV in lung CT AI work is optimally chosen to include only the lungs to keep the DFOV as small as possible, typically 32 cm. It is also important to use the same DFOV and matrix size when multiple scans are obtained over time on the patient. It should be noted that all scanners can reconstruct the acquired 1D projections using various DFOV sizes without exposing the patient to additional radiation. For example, there can be one reconstruction for lung CT AI work, 32 cm DFOV, and a larger DFOV to be sure to assess all of the chest wall structures, 45 cm DFOV.

Hounsfield Units and the CT Voxel

After the CT image reconstruction process is completed, we have a 3D representation of the thorax containing millions of voxels. Each voxel is assigned a value that represents the average x-ray photon linear attenuation coefficient of the tissue contained within the voxel. These are small numbers with the units cm^{-1} and symbol μ. The linear attenuation coefficient of liquid water, μ_{water}, using 50 keV photons is 0.214 cm^{-1}.[5] The linear attenuation of dry air, μ_{air}, using 50 keV photons is 0.000290.[5]

Since the beginning of CT scanning in the early 1970s, there has been a desire to express these linear attenuation coefficients in a manner that is simple and easy to understand. This resulted in the Hounsfield unit (HU) scale, named after Sir Godfrey Hounsfield who invented the first human x-ray CT scanner in 1972.[1,2]

The Hounsfield Unit is defined using the linear attenuation coefficients of air, water, and the tissue in question, as follows:

$$HU = 1000 \times ((\mu_{tissue} - \mu_{water})/(\mu_{water} - \mu_{air}))$$

Where HU is the tissue density in Hounsfield Units. The Hounsfield scale range assigns a value to air of −1000 HU and a value to water of 0 HU. The scale typically runs from −1000 HU to 3095 HU for a 12-bit CT scanner.[1] The range of densities in the normal lung range from −1000 HU to 40 HU. The normal lung is comprised of 80% air and 20% tissue, so it is not surprising that the normal lung density range is −843 HU in adult males and −824 HU in adult females.[13]

It should be noted that tissue density measured in HU numbers can be converted to a more familiar measure of tissue density, mass per unit volume in units of grams per liter, by adding 1000 to the HU value. This assumes the density of air is 0 g/L and the density of water is 1000 g/L. For example, the HU number for water is 0, and if we add 1000 we get the density of water, which is 1000 g/L or 1 g/cm³.

Visually Display of Lung Images

The next step is deciding how best to visually interact with the 3D digital images of the thorax that contains the lung. The most common method is to view the entire anatomy contained in the DFOV. This includes structures with air density, such as air in the trachea with a density of −1000 HU, to cortical bone with a density of 1800 HU. Here we assume a high-quality medical display capable of displaying 2048 grey levels with a luminance range of 0.5 to 2000 cd/m².[14] If the range of CT numbers is assumed to be 4096, or 12-bits of information, then how does the human eye evaluate the anatomy when the human eye at best can distinguish 900 shades of grey on a state of the art medical display?[14] The answer is that we look at a subset of the grey levels and, as a result, we need to look at images that are optimized to look at lung tissue, soft tissues, or bony structures. Here we are interested in looking at the human lung, so we are interested in looking at CT density values between −1000 HU to 40 HU. The range, or window width (WW), of HU values is typically set at 1500 HU instead of 1040 HU for viewing x-ray CT images of the lung. The wider WW decreases image contrast, which, in the case of the x-ray CT images of the lung, yields a more acceptable image contrast. A WW of 1040 is selected to assess very subtle differences in tissue density. The mid-point of this 1040-1500 scale or window level (WL) is usually set between −500 and −600 HU. Fig. 2.12 shows an axial x-ray CT image of the thorax with different WW and WL settings. There are other enhanced visualizations available to assess

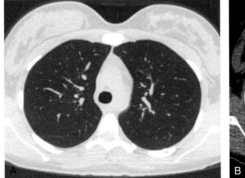 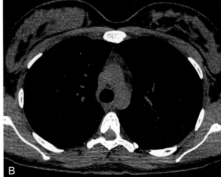

Fig. 2.12 2D axial image of the thorax with WW = 1500 and WL = −500, which is optimized for looking at the lungs **(A)**, and WW = 350 and WL = 50, which is optimized to look at the soft tissue structures in the mediastinum and chest wall **(B)**.

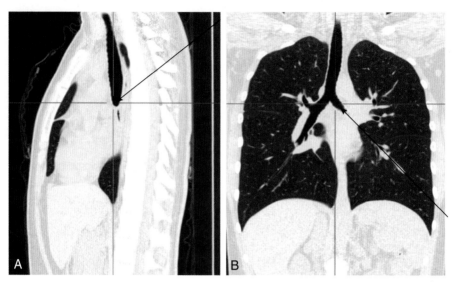

Fig. 2.13 Example of multiplanar lung CT images of the thorax in the sagittal **(A)** and coronal **(B)** planes using WW = 1500 and WL = −500. This is the same normal CT study as Fig. 2.12. The intersection of the horizontal and vertical lines in each image *(arrows)* are identifying the same CT voxel, which is near the bifurcation of the trachea into the right and left main-stem bronchi.

the human lung, including multiplanar reformatted images in the sagittal and coronal planes (Fig. 2.13). There are also maximum intensity projections (MIPS) and minimum intensity projections (MinIPS) available in axial, coronal, and sagittal planes. The MIPS help in identifying lung nodules separate from lung blood vessels. The MinIPS are helpful for identifying air-containing structures, such as emphysema, and normal or dilated airway lumens. Two new lung CT image formats that have recently been introduced by the lung CT AI company VIDA Diagnostics Inc. in Coralville, Iowa. These new image formats are topographic multiplanar images that are optimized to view the airway tree, airway tMPR (Fig. 2.14), and the subpleural space of the lungs, subpleural images.

We will use representative examples of lung CT images in this book that visually show the lung disease features that are being assessed by corresponding lung CT AI methods.

Quantitative CT Metrics

There are a number of quantitative x-ray CT metrics that have been developed in lung CT AI studies of normal and diseased lung structure and function, and these will be discussed in Chapters 4 through 7. These include measurements of lung volume, lung tissue intensity, lung tissue texture, air trapping, and lung tissue biomechanics.

CT Scanning Protocols

CT scanning protocols of the lung are designed to achieve accurate and precise CT images of the lung, with the needed spatial and contrast resolution, using the smallest amount of ionizing x-ray radiation dose to the scanned tissues. These CT scanning

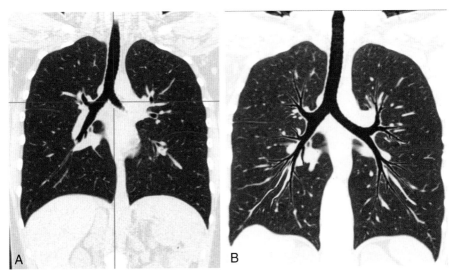

Fig. 2.14 Normal coronal image of the thorax **(A)** and a corresponding airway topographic MPR image that is optimized to show the trachea, main-stem bronchi, lobar bronchi, and segmental bronchi in a single image **(B)**.

protocols are very detailed and are critical to the field of lung CT AI. The important elements of these CT protocols will be discussed in Chapter 3 and will build on the discussions in this chapter. These CT protocols can be pre-programmed into the current generation of CT scanners available in the 2020s. This greatly simplifies the CT scanning process for clinical patients and research subjects.

X-ray CT Radiation Dose

The differential absorption and scattering of the x-ray beam photons provide the means to generate transmission x-ray CT images previously described. Unfortunately, the x-ray photons that undergo photoelectric absorption and Compton scattering deposit energy in the tissues can damage DNA molecules.[15–17] The DNA damage is proportional to the energy that is transferred from the incoming x-ray photon to the kinetic energy of free electrons. At the level of x-ray radiation dose given for a typical chest CT scan, 17 mGy, the damage to the DNA increases the stochastic risk of developing cancer in a linear fashion with increasing x-ray dose.[17] The kinetic energy of these free electrons that are deposited per unit mass of tissue is referred to as the absorbed dose and is expressed as energy in Joules deposited per kilogram of tissue and its SI unit is the gray (Gy).[15] The higher the absorbed radiation dose in the tissues, the greater the potential for DNA damage. The mass-energy absorption coefficient of the x-ray photons times the energy fluence of the x-ray photons equals the absorbed dose to the tissues.[5] The x-ray beam intensity largely determines the signal-to-noise ratio in the x-ray CT images and also largely determines the ionizing radiation dose that the patient receives from an x-ray CT scan. The ALARA (As Low As Reasonably Achievable) principle guides physicians in deciding how much radiation dose to give a patient or research subject for an x-ray CT scan of the thorax.[16] The ALARA principle means we should give only as much radiation as necessary to achieve the goal of the x-ray CT scan.[16] It is important to follow the ALARA principle when designing lung CT scanning protocols.

$CTDI_{vol}$ is a method that is used to try and quantitate the absorbed radiation dose to the thorax that a patient receives from a CT scan of the thorax.[15] The units of the $CTDI_{vol}$ are Gys. A typical $CTDI_{vol}$ dose from an x-ray CT scan of the thorax is 17 mGy. A low-dose CT scan is considered one in which the $CTDI_{vol}$ is less than 3 mGy.[18] The $CTDI_{vol}$ value is reported by the x-ray CT scanner.

The length of the scan (L) in cm in the z-axis is also important to take into consideration.[15] The typical L value for a tall adult male is 30 cm. The dose length product (DLP) is the product of the $CTDI_{vol}$ multiplied by L and has units of mGy-cm. The DLP is also reported by the CT scanner; the $CTDI_{vol}$ and DLP are included in the x-ray report.

The effective dose for a chest CT scan is a stochastic method of assessing what the whole-body radiation dose to a "generic patient" would have to be to impart the same risks of inducing cancer as the absorbed dose to the chest using a given $CTDI_{vol}$, L, and conversion factor (k). k varies by the body part that is being scanned. The chest CT has a k factor equal to 0.014 mSv/mGy-cm.[15] The effective dose can be calculated using the following formula:

$$E = CTDI_{vol} \times DLP \times k$$

Using a $CTDI_{vol}$ of 17 mGy, L of 30 cm, and k of 0.014 mSv/mGy-cm from a typical chest CT scan, the corresponding whole-body effective dose for a generic patient would be 7 mSv. The effective dose is an important parameter in developing lung CT scanning protocols for lung CT AI research and clinical scanning. The effective dose estimate for an x-ray CT scanning protocol can be used to convey risk to the patient or research subject by comparing this whole-body effective dose to the average yearly background whole-body radiation effective dose in the United States, which is 3.1 mSv.[19] The $CTDI_{vol}$ in mGy, and not the effective CT dose in mSv, is used to express the radiation dose to an individual patient.[15] The size-specific dose estimate (SSDE) can be used to improve upon the $CTDI_{vol}$ as a measure of the x-ray radiation dose that an individual patient receives from an x-ray CT scan.[15] AAPM Reports 204 and 246 describe how to calculate the SSDE given the $CTDI_{vol}$ using the following formula:

$$SSDE = f_{wed} \times CTDI_{vol}$$

where f_{wed} is a size-specific conversion factor based on the water equivalent diameter (wed) of the patient.[20,21] The $CTDI_{vol}$ underestimates the radiation dose, especially in smaller patients, and the SSDE can provide a more accurate measure of individual patient dose than the $CTDI_{vol}$. The input parameters to determine f_{wed} for a chest CT are the maximum AP and Lateral dimensions of the patient's chest.[20,21] These are used to calculate an effective diameter:

$$diameter_{effective} = \left((AP\ diameter) \times (Lateral\ Diameter)\right)^{1/2}$$

AAPM Report 206 Table 1D can be used to calculate f_{wed} if the effective diameter is known. The value of f_{wed} for an effective diameter of 16 cm is 2.06 and the f_{wed} for an effective diameter of 32 cm is 1.14. SSDE is more than twice the value of the $CTDI_{vol}$

for the smaller effective diameter. Further discussions of SSDE go beyond the scope of this book, the interested reader is referred to the literature.[15,20,21]

Brief History of X-ray CT

In this section of the chapter, we will highlight how x-ray CT of the lungs have gone from very large voxels, low signal-to-noise ratio, long scanning times with higher radiation dose to very small voxels, higher signal-to-noise ratio, and very short scanning times with lower radiation dose. The first CT scans of the lungs generated digital numerical values that were assigned to the volume elements, or voxels, making up the CT images of the lungs. The numerical values represent the x-ray linear attenuation coefficients of the tissues. A simple rescaling of these linear attenuation coefficients was done to generate a linear scale expressed in Hounsfield Units (HU) that was more intuitive.[1,2]

The complete three-dimensional (3D) CT scan of the lung is built up by reconstructing consecutive 2D images of the lung. The first CT scanners would typically acquire one or two images per rotation of the x-ray tube and detector around the patient. There would then be an interscan delay while the scanning table on which the patient was lying supine would move on the z-axis and the x-ray tube and detector were moved back to their starting position for the next scan. This completed the acquisition of the 1D projections to reconstruct a 2D image of the patient at a particular z-coordinate. The patient would be moved in the direction of his or her head or feet to be ready for the next 2D image. This process of scanning the patient, interscan delay, and moving the patient are referred to as axial mode CT imaging. This process would be repeated until the entire thorax was scanned or, depending on the capabilities of the early CT scanner and the clinical question that needed to be answered, a subset scanned.

THE FIRST HEAD AND BODY CT SCANNERS – 1971 TO 1975 (EMI, ACTA, OHIO NUCLEAR)

The first human head CT scanner was developed by Sir Godfrey Hounsfield at EMI over a period of 6 years, with the first head CT scan performed in 1971.[2,22] Hounsfield recognized the ability of x-ray CT to distinguish small differences in tissue density; 0.5%, would give it abilities that existing projection radiography could not match, for example separating normal brain tissue from a brain tumor, even though the spatial resolution of the EMI Mark 1 CT scanner needed to be far less than the existing spatial resolution of projection radiography, 0.5 mm, to keep the computation time reasonable for clinical practice.[22] The first head CT scan of a human brain was of a woman with a brain tumor and was performed in 1971. When the scan was displayed, Hounsfield is quoted as saying "My God, it does work—I can see the tumor just as I had always hoped".[22] Hounsfield was right, and the first head CT scans represented a revolutionary breakthrough in noninvasive diagnostic medical imaging. This first CT scanner could scan the human head, but not the body. This was because it required a "water bath" around the patient's head to even out the attenuation of the highly collimated x-ray beam that was used to acquire the head images. The water bath was necessary to reduce the intensity range of the x-ray photons to match the detector response characteristics more closely. The reconstruction method was an algebraic reconstruction technique

(ART), as opposed to a filtered back projection method. The need for a water bath made it impractical to scan the thorax and abdomen of a patient. The EMI Mark 1 x-ray CT scanner was introduced at the 1972 Annual Meeting of the Radiological Society of North America and orders were taken.[22] EMI was the only vendor in 1972, but by the 1973 Annual Meeting of the RSNA, Ohio Nuclear had announced the development of a clone of the EMI Mark 1 scanner with scan times reduced from 5 minutes to 2 minutes, and image matrix size increased to 120 × 120. EMI was still selling the Mark 1 but announced the improved Mark 2 scanner at the 1973 RSNA meeting. During this time, Georgetown University sent Robert Ledley to EMI in the United Kingdom to look into acquiring an EMI Mark 1 head CT scanner for the university.[22] Upon his return, Ledley convinced Georgetown University that he could develop a head and body CT scanner, and obtained approval to do this. Ledley was able to develop his new whole-body CT scanner in just 18 months.[22]

The first whole-body x-ray CT scanner was the Automatic Computerized Transverse Axial (ACTA) Scanner. It was developed by Robert Ledley, MS, DDS, at Georgetown University in Washington, DC, in 1973 (Patent No. 3,922,552).[23-25] Robert Ledley was a biophysicist and dentist at Georgetown University who reported the first CT images of the lungs in 1975 in the journal *Radiology*.[26] It is helpful to go through the components of this scanner to see where x-ray chest CT technology began, so as to better appreciate the technical advancements that have led to the current highly capable chest x-ray CT scanners of the 2020 s.

The ACTA scanner consisted of a gantry that housed the x-ray tube and two x-ray detectors, with the patient positioned on a translatable table located in the center of the gantry aperture between the x-ray tube and the x-ray detectors. The x-ray tube beam was collimated to form a pencil beam that exposed 7.5 mm of two separate x-ray detectors, with each detector separated by 3 mm. This would be described as a multidetector x-ray CT scanner since two adjacent CT images were obtained for each 180-degree rotation of the x-ray tube and x-ray detector array. The x-ray detectors were composed of a sodium iodide crystal attached to a photomultiplier tube. The x-rays would produce visible light when they interacted with the iodide atoms in the sodium iodide crystal and the photomultiplier tube would amplify the light signal. Then, this signal would be digitized and stored in the computer. The sampling window was 5 ms to measure the x-ray intensity at one point of the projection. The x-ray tube and crystal assembly would translate in a line across the patient making 160 of these 5-ms measurements to obtain a 1D projection of the object being scanned. The x-ray tube and detector array would then rotate 1 degree and the process would repeat itself. This process was done until the x-ray and detector array had rotated 180 degrees around the patient. This produced 180 projections of the patient. The combination of each 160 points collected for each projection, multiplied by 180 projections, would result in a total of 28,800 measurements for each reconstructed 2D image of the object being scanned. The 180 projections of the object were then reconstructed using the Fourier slice theorem.[23] The reconstructed 2D image was made up of 25,600 points forming a 160 × 160 image matrix.[23] The spatial resolution of the CT images in the z-direction was 7.5 mm. The x–y resolution was 1.5 mm. There were two scanning modes available: short pass, 24 cm, and long pass, 48 cm. This would be similar to the SFOV, as described previously. In the long pass, the x-ray tube and detector array would linearly translate 48 cm across the patient to obtain one complete 1D projection and was used for scans of the thorax, abdomen, and pelvis. This process would be repeated 180 times at 1-degree increments. This scan would take 6 minutes to obtain two 2D axial images of the thorax. The short pass scan mode was used to scan the head, neck, and extremities. There was doubt as to how useful the CT scans of the thorax would be given the 6-minute scan time to obtain two images—total examination time to scan a 30-cm adult thorax would be at least 90 minutes. The respiratory and cardiac motion was well-tolerated and the CT images presented an average appearance over the time of the scan. The first images of the thorax showed a lung cancer nodule in the left lung; the trachea, transverse aorta, and superior vena cava were identified, along with the muscles and bones in the chest wall.[23]

It can be seen from the detailed description of the first whole-body x-ray CT scanner that certain design features would be retained and others improved upon; if the goal was collecting more projection data, in a shorter period, with higher spatial resolution, while also maintaining the high intrinsic contrast resolution of x-ray CT compared to x-ray projection radiography. The basic layout of a gantry housing the x-ray tube and corresponding detector array with the patient positioned between the x-ray beam and detector is retained, along with having the patient lay quietly on a table that traverses the central aperture of the CT gantry. Improvements that needed to be made over the EMI Mark 1 and ACTA CT scanner designs included increased size of the x-ray beam with corresponding increases in the overall size of the detector array, increased number of detector elements, increased speed at which 1D projections are obtained, and improvements in electronics and computing power.

RAPID EVOLUTION OF CT SCANNER DESIGNS

Between 1973 and 1983, there was intense competition between manufacturers and rapid evolution of whole-body x-ray CT scanner designs.[22] During this rapid phase of advances in x-ray CT scanner technology, four different x-ray tube detector array arrangements were developed. These were distinguished by different x-ray beam geometry, x-ray detector array size, and the type, size, and number of x-ray detector elements, and how the x-ray tube and corresponding x-ray detector array rotated around the patient.[1,22] The initial EMI Mark 1 head CT scanner and the ACTA whole-body CT scanner were termed a pencil beam translate-rotate generation one design (Fig. 2.5). Second-generation CT scanners were termed broad parallel beam translate-rotate CT scanners (Fig. 2.5). Third-generation CT scanners were termed fan-beam rotate/rotate CT scanners (Fig. 2.5). Fourth-generation CT scanners were termed fan-beam rotate/stationary CT scanners (Fig. 2.5). The scan time to acquire one 2D image of the thorax had decreased from 6 minutes to 5 seconds by 1983. This process would have to be repeated multiple times to scan the entire human thorax. This axial scanning method was used by most x-ray CT scanners until 1990.

The winning design that was firmly established by 1983, among the four generations previously described, was the third-generation CT scanners where the x-ray tube and detector rotated around the patient in a circular arc.[22] The two most successful manufacturers in 1983 were GE and Siemens.[1,22] The third-generation fan-beam x-ray tube rotates in a circle and the corresponding x-ray detector also rotates in a circle. Typically, this type of CT scanner has a SFOV of 50 cm and a distance from the x-ray tube anode to the isocenter of the CT gantry of 50 cm.[1] The optimal fan angle, alpha, for this arrangement can be calculated from the following formula[1]:

$$SFOV = 25 \times \sin\left(alpha/2\right)$$

Using this formula, if the SFOV = 50 cm, then the optimal fan beam angle alpha is equal to 60-degrees.[1] The fan-shaped x-ray beam subtended 60 degrees at the curved detector array (Fig. 2.4). The patient would hold their breath while one image was obtained, then would breathe again. The entire examination would take 10 minutes or more, depending on how frequently the patient could perform repeated breath holds. This process was very time-consuming and prevented acquiring a 3D set of lung images obtained during a single breath-hold. The axial scanning sequence was typically performed using 10-mm slice thickness at 10-mm intervals to cover the entire lung. The contiguous 10-mm slice CT images were used to detect and assess the size of lung nodules, or the extent of emphysema or pneumonia. The resolution of the 10-mm slice acquisition was low when compared to modern CT scanners being used in the 2020 s. The beamwidth needed to be decreased using different strategies for narrowing the x-ray beam to obtain images with higher z-axis resolution (if additional high-resolution CT (HRCT) images of the lung were needed), which required rescanning the patient using a slice thickness of 1 to 2 mm at 10- to 20-mm intervals to keep the x-ray dose from becoming excessive. The next big breakthrough in CT scanner technology did not happen for almost 10 years when the single detector array helical, or spiral, CT scanner was developed.

MODERATE-RESOLUTION WHOLE LUNG ACQUISITION IN A SINGLE BREATH—SPIRAL CT SCANNER

The spiral CT scanner was a major advancement, when compared to the previous axial CT scanners, because the patient could be scanned continuously. The first reports of a spiral CT scanner were published in 1990.[27–29] This dramatically reduced the time it took to scan an entire thorax. For the first time, both lungs could be scanned in a single breath-hold.[30] The idea here is that the x-ray tube and detector array are continuously rotating around the subject using a slip ring design of the CT scanner gantry. The patient can then be continuously transported on a table through the CT gantry aperture while the x-ray tube and detector continuously rotate around the patient. The x-ray tube and detector array in the reference frame of the patient, trace out a spiral, or helical pattern, hence the name, spiral or helical CT (Fig. 2.7). These two names mean the same thing, but there was some controversy as to which should be used.[31] We will use the term spiral CT in this book. The amount of scan data acquired per unit time generated during spiral scans was much greater than the slower axial scanning process of rotate once, rewind the x-ray tube and detector, and move the table. This meant that the electronic components that capture the detector data, digitize it, and transport it off the scanner into the computer needed much higher performance than those used for earlier axial mode only CT scanners. Many new advances in x-ray tube power, x-ray detector resolution and sensitivity, detector electronics, and computer hardware and software were needed to generate and transmit the large amount of digital data that spiral CT scanning demanded. The need for continuous spinning of the x-ray tube and detector array in spiral CT scanning required the third-generation design (where the x-ray tube and x-ray detector array rotated together around the patient inside of another stationary concentric cylinder) and this design has continued into the 2020s. The single detector array spiral CT scanners would still typically select a slice thickness of 10 mm for the contiguous images of the lungs. Repeat axial scanning, with 1- to 2-mm collimation at 10- to 20-mm intervals, was still necessary for high-resolution CT images of the lungs to better assess emphysema and pulmonary fibrosis.

HIGH-RESOLUTION LUNG CT IN A SINGLE BREATH FOR ALL PATIENTS: MULTIDETECTOR SPIRAL CT SCANNERS

The next major breakthrough in CT scanner design was the the Multdetector Spiral CT (MDCT) scanner that effectively acquired multiple 2D axial images of the lungs with each 360-degree rotation of the x-ray tube by using a two-dimensional detector array. "Multiple detector" is a somewhat confusing term because the previous spiral and axial CT scanners had multiple detectors, but they were all in the x–y plane and at the same z-axis coordinate of the patient. The one-dimensional detector arrays acquired a single image for each 360-degree rotation of the x-ray tube. The 2D detector arrays began with two detector rows on the z-axis of the patient and then subsequent advances led to 4 rows, 8 rows, 16 rows, 32 rows, 64 rows, 128 rows, 256 rows, and more. The 2D detector effectively acquires multiple adjacent 2D images with each 360-degree rotation of the x-ray tube. When 64-row MDCT scanners became available in the mid to late 2000s, the time to scan a 30 cm (z-axis) lung was greatly improved. A typical protocol would specify 0.5 second rotation time, 64 detectors × 0.625 mm detector width for a beamwidth of 40 mm, and a pitch of 1. The scan time was 7.5 seconds and would generate up to 480 0.625 mm thick high-resolution 2D axial images of the lung. This was a very important advancement in the assessment of lung disease since patients with chronic lung disease are short of breath and it is difficult for them to hold their breath for more than 12 seconds. The 64-row MDCT scanners are often the minimum necessary for acquiring high-resolution 3D images of the lungs in patients with significant shortness of breath due to lung disease. For the purposes of applying AI software to segment the lungs from the rest of the thoracic anatomy and to extract quantitative metrics of lung disease, high-resolution 3D images with submillimeter resolution in all three spatial coordinate axis x, y, and z, is optimal.

We will use the technical details we discussed in this chapter in Chapter 3 to build lung CT AI CT scanning protocols that are optimized for quantitative CT work using modern 64-row or greater MDCT scanners.

References

1. Bushberg JT, Seibert JA, Leidholdt Jr EM, Boone JM. *Computed Tomography. The Essential Physics of Medical Imaging.* 3rd ed. Philadelphia, PA: Wolters Kluwer, Lippincott Williams & Wilkins; 2012:312–374.
2. Hounsfield GN. Nobel Award address. Computed medical imaging. *Med Phys.* 1980;7(4):283–290.
3. Newell Jr JD, Fuld MK, Allmendinger T, Sieren JP, Chan KS, Guo J, et al. Very low-dose (0.15 mGy) chest CT protocols using the COPDGene 2 test object and a third-generation

dual-source CT scanner with corresponding third-generation iterative reconstruction software. *Invest Radiol.* 2015;50(1):40–45.

4. Bushberg JT, Seibert JA, Leidholdt Jr EM, Boone JM. *Radiation and the Atom. The Essential Physics of Medical Imaging.* 3rd ed. Philadelphia, PA: Wolters Kluwer, Lippincott Williams & Wilkins; 2012:18–32.

5. Bushberg JT, Seibert JA, Leidholdt Jr EM, Boone JM. *Interaction of Radiation with Matter. The Essential Physics of Medical Imaging.* 3rd ed. Philadelphia, PA: Wolters Kluwer, Lippincott Williams & Wilkins; 2012:33–59.

6. Bushberg JT, Seibert JA, Leidholdt Jr EM, Boone JM. *X-ray Production, X-ray Tubes, and X-ray Generators. The Essential Physics of Medical Imaging.* 3rd ed. Philadelphia, PA: Wolters Kluwer, Lippincott Williams & Wilkins; 2012:171–206.

7. Chemicool. Tungsten Element Facts 2020. Accessed April 20,2022. https://www.chemicool.com/elements/tungsten.html.

8. Danielsson M, Persson M, Sjolin M. Photon-counting x-ray detectors for CT. *Phys Med Biol.* 2021;66(3):03TR1.

9. Toth T, Ge Z, Daly MP. The influence of patient centering on CT dose and image noise. *Med Phys.* 2007;34(7):3093–3101.

10. Saltybaeva N, Alkadhi H. Vertical off-centering affects organ dose in chest CT: Evidence from Monte Carlo simulations in anthropomorphic phantoms. *Med Phys.* 2017;44(11):5697–5704.

11. Sukupova L, Vedlich D, Jiru F. Consequences of the Patient's Mis-centering on the Radiation Dose and Image Quality in CT Imaging – Phantom and Clinical Study. *Univers J Med Sci.* 2016;4(3):102–107.

12. Stiller W. Basics of iterative reconstruction methods in computed tomography: A vendor-independent overview. *Eur J Radiol.* 2018;109:147–154.

13. Kim SS, Jin GY, Li YZ, Lee JE, Shin HS. CT Quantification of Lungs and Airways in Normal Korean Subjects. *Korean J Radiol.* 2017;18(4):739–748.

14. Kimpe T, Tuytschaever T. Increasing the number of gray shades in medical display systems—how much is enough? *J Digit Imaging.* 2007;20(4):422–432.

15. Bushberg JT, Seibert JA, Leidholdt Jr EM, Boone JM. *X-ray Dosimetry in Projection Imaging and Computed Tomography. The Essential Physics of Medical Imaging.* 3rd ed. Philadelphia, PA: Wolters Kluwer, Lippincott Williams & Wilkins; 2012:375–401.

16. Bushberg JT, Seibert JA, Leidholdt Jr EM, Boone JM. *Radiation Protection. The Essential Physics of Medical Imaging.* 3rd ed. Philadelphia, PA: Wolters Kluwer, Lippincott Williams & Wilkins; 2012:837–909.

17. Bushberg JT, Seibert JA, Leidholdt Jr EM, Boone JM. *Radiation Biology. The Essential Physics of Medical Imaging.* 3rd ed. Philadelphia, PA: Wolters Kluwer, Lippincott Williams & Wilkins; 2012:751–836.

18. AAPM. Lung Cancer Screening CT Protocols Version 5.1. 13 September 2019. Accessed April 20, 2022 https://www.aapm.org/pubs/ctprotocols/documents/lungcancerscreeningct.pdf.

19. Bushberg JT, Seibert JA, Leidholdt Jr EM, Boone JM. *Radiation Dose: Perspectives and Comparisons. The Essential Physics of Medical Imaging.* 3rd ed. Philadelphia, PA: Wolters Kluwer, Lippincott Williams & Wilkins; 2012:998–1004.

20. AAPM. *Size Specific Dose Estimates (SSDE) in Pediatric and Adult Body CT Examinations.* College Park, MD: AAPM; 2011:204.

21. AAPM *Estimating Patient Organ Dose with Computed Tomography: A Review of Present Methodology and Requried DICOM Information.* College Park, MD: AAPM; 2019:246.

22. Robb WL. Perspective on the First 10 Years of the CT Scanner Industry. *Academic Radiology.* 2003;10(7):756–760.

23. Ledley RS, Di Chiro G, Luessenhop AJ, Twigg HL. Computerized transaxial x-ray tomography of the human body. *Science.* 1974;186(4160):207–212.
24. Ledley RS, Wilson JB, Golab T, Rotolo LS. The ACTA-scanner: the whole body computerized transaxial tomograph. *Comput Biol Med.* 1974;4(2):145–155.
25. Sittig DF, Ash JS, Ledley RS. The story behind the development of the first whole-body computerized tomography scanner as told by Robert S. Ledley. *J Am Med Inform Assoc.* 2006;13(5):465–469.
26. Schellinger D, Di Chiro G, Axelbaum SP, Twigg HL, Ledley RS. Early clinical experience with the ACTA scanner. *Radiology.* 1975;114(2):257–261.
27. Kalender WA, Seissler W, Klotz E, Vock P. Spiral volumetric CT with single-breath-hold technique, continuous transport, and continuous scanner rotation. *Radiology.* 1990;176(1):181–183.
28. Kalender WA, Vock P, Polacin A, Soucek M. Spiral-CT: a new technique for volumetric scans. I. Basic principles and methodology. *Rontgenpraxis.* 1990;43(9):323–330.
29. Soucek M, Vock P, Daepp M, Kalender WA. Spiral-CT: a new technique for volumetric scans. II. *Potential clinical applications. Rontgenpraxis.* 1990;43(10):365–375.
30. Vock P, Soucek M, Daepp M, Kalender WA. Lung: spiral volumetric CT with single-breath-hold technique. *Radiology.* 1990;176(3):864–867.
31. Kalender WA. Spiral or helical CT: right or wrong? *Radiology.* 1994;193(2):583.

CHAPTER 3

X-ray CT Scanning Protocols for Lung CT AI Applications

In this chapter we will discuss the elements of chest CT scanning protocols that are optimized for lung CT AI applications.[1-7] These lung CT AI applications can be divided into visual CT (VCT) applications, where the analysis of the lung CT images is done by an expert imaging physician, and quantitative CT (QCT) applications, where the image analysis is done by AI. The focus of this book is on QCT AI applications, so we will focus primarily on the elements of QCT scanning protocols and how the elements of these protocols were developed over time. The technology requirements for QCT of the lung go beyond those that are necessary for VCT of the lung, though there are many elements of a VCT scanning protocol that are also common in a QCT scanning protocol.

Visual and quantitative chest CT scanning protocols need to address ionizing radiation dose using the ALARA principle (see Chapter 2). The radiation dose needs to be kept as low as possible while providing the CT image quality necessary to achieve the goals of the CT study. The goals of a VCT study may not need as demanding a CT scanning protocol as a QCT study. It is important to not administer more ionizing radiation dose than is necessary to achieve the objectives of the study and to keep in mind that the effective dose of chest CT studies should be in the range of 1 to 10 mSv, depending on the application. Low-dose CT studies are defined as those that have an effective dose less than 1 mSv. Low-dose studies should be done where the objectives of the study can be obtained with a low-dose CT scanning protocol.

Additional elements of visual and quantitative chest CT scanning protocols include x-ray tube peak voltage (kVp) and tube current time product (mAs), as well as x-ray tube current and voltage modulation, x-ray beam collimation and additional filtration, pitch, positioning the patient at the isocenter of the CT gantry, total time for the examination, supine versus prone positioning of the patient on the CT scanner table, lung volume used for the scan, and making sure the patient is coached to the selected lung volume, SFOV, DFOV, reconstruction method (FBP vs IR), and reconstruction kernel (Box 3.1). It is important to have a quality control (QC) program for both VCT and QCT that includes the use of CT phantoms, which are inanimate objects that simulate various material densities and structures contained in the human thorax to routinely determine if the CT scanner is working properly. There is also the need to decide how long the projection data is kept on the scanner so additional CT image reconstructions can be done if there is something that was done incorrectly in the image reconstruction process. The transfer of CT data to different sites via intranets and internets needs to be worked out, too.

BOX 3.1 ■ Lung CT Scanning Protocol Elements Common to Visual and Quantitative Lung CT

1. Radiation dose adheres to "As Low As Reasonably Achievable" (ALARA) Principle
2. Routine quality control procedures
   a. X-ray CT quality control phantoms
   b. X-ray CT projection data retained for short period of time (e.g., 48 hours)
3. X-ray tube peak voltage (kV)
4. X-ray tube current time product (mAs)
5. X-ray tube focal spot, filters, and collimation
6. X-ray tube current modulation
7. X-ray tube rotation time, CT table velocity and resultant pitch
8. Patient positioning
   a. Isocenter
   b. Supine versus prone
9. Scan field of view (SFOV), display field of view (DFOV)
   a. Size of reconstruction matrix (e.g., 512 × 512, 1024 × 1024)
10. Breathing the patient to the proper lung volume
    a. Total lung capacity (TLC)–deep inspiration
    b. Functional residual capacity (FRC)–normal passive expiration
    c. Residual volume (RV)–deep expiration
11. CT reconstruction method
    a. Reconstruction kernel
    b. Filtered back projection (FBP)
    c. Iterative reconstruction (IR)
    d. Deep machine learning reconstruction
12. Axial CT image reconstruction width and interval
13. Transmission, storage, and display of CT images

The quantitative CT scanning protocols that drive lung CT AI have been developed to try and address the issue of generating the most precise and accurate voxel size and CT numbers (HU) assigned to each voxel within the CT lung images, and to maintain the precision and accuracy of the CT voxels contained in the lung CT images over time and on different CT scanner make and models. We will review how the current quantitative CT scanning protocols were developed.

Early Work in the Development of QCT Scanning Protocols

Dirksen et al. reported in 1999 that quantitative CT using the 15th percentile point of the lung density histogram showed decreased progression of alpha-1 antitrypsin deficiency (A1AD) induced emphysema in A1AD patients who were receiving monthly intravenous augmentation therapy with human alpha-AT.[8] The quantitative CT results were much more sensitive than monitoring decreases in airflow measured by using the forced expiratory volume in one second, FEV1. This was a turning point in the development of lung CT AI using quantitative CT metrics, such as the 15th percentile method, because now quantitative lung CT was doing something noninvasively that visual lung CT and pulmonary physiological measures of lung function could not do.

WORKSHOP: QUANTITATIVE COMPUTED TOMOGRAPHY SCANNING IN LONGITUDINAL STUDIES OF EMPHYSEMA

The excitement around Dirksen's paper in 1999 led to the Alpha-1 Foundation organizing a workshop entitled "Quantitative Computed Tomography Scanning in Longitudinal Studies of Emphysema" that took place February 2 and 3, 2001.[4,8] The workshop brought together experts in thoracic radiology, pulmonology, and lung pathology to explore current state-of-the-art CT imaging used to quantitate pulmonary emphysema, and to discuss the feasibility of using quantitative lung CT image data as a primary endpoint in drug trials designed to assess new treatments for A1AD.[4] The primary goal of the workshop was to develop a consensus on the optimal parameters to be included in a quantitative CT scanning protocol that would be recommended for randomized, double-blind, multicenter drug trials for the treatment of A1AD.

Can X-ray CT Detect and Quantify Pulmonary Emphysema?

Pulmonary emphysema is defined as "abnormal permanent enlargement of air spaces distal to the terminal bronchioles, accompanied by destruction of their walls and without obvious fibrosis."[4,9] The workshop pointed out that the increase in the size of the airspace of the lung alveoli and the decrease in tissue mass due to destruction of the alveolar walls would cause a decrease in tissue density, g/mL. As was pointed out in Chapter 2, the CT numbers assigned to the individual voxels of the lung CT images correspond closely to the density of lung tissue. Therefore, CT scanning should be able to assess the presence and extent of pulmonary emphysema both visually and quantitatively.

Single Versus Multiple Detector Row CT Scanners

At the time of the workshop, multiple-detector spiral CT scanners (MDCT), as described in Chapter 2, were increasing in number and had advantages over the single-detector spiral CT (SDCT) scanners that preceded them. It was pointed out that the MDCT scanners were preferable to SDCT scanners in the QCT assessment of emphysema. This is because the greater the number of detector rows in the z-axis of the patient, the faster the entire lungs could be scanned. This is especially important in patients that are short of breath due to their underlying emphysema. Four-, 8-, and 16-row MDCT scanners with a detector width of 1.0 to 1.25 mm could obtain high-resolution images of the entire lungs in 25 to 30 seconds, 10 seconds, and 5 seconds, respectively.[4] Sixteen-row MDCT scanners would be preferable, if available.

It was also recognized that for longitudinal studies, the same CT scanner model should be used at the different study time points for a given patient throughout the course of the study. If different CT scanner models were going to be used in a study for the same study patient, CT phantoms need to be used to verify that the different CT scanner models had equivalent spatial and density resolution.[7]

Constant and Optimal X-ray Tube Peak Kilovoltage, mAs, and Radiation Dose

The x-ray tube peak voltage and x-ray tube current time product were discussed in the workshop and, given the MDCT technology at the time, it was agreed that the peak x-ray tube voltage should be between 120 and 140 kV and the same x-ray tube peak voltage should be used for all subjects in a given study.[4] This is because the x-ray tube peak voltage determines the x-ray photon beam spectrum coming from the anode of the x-ray tube. Additional x-ray beam shaping and filtration placed in front of the x-ray tube, but before the patient, were not specifically addressed. The majority of the workshop participants favored setting the tube current time product between 80 and 100 mAs to provide acceptable image-to-noise ratio in the lung, while greater values would increase the ionizing radiation dose to the subject/patient without realizing any additional benefit.[4] Twenty mAs was suggested as the minimum possible for a particular CT scanner model and CT scanning protocol.[4] The recommended dose should follow the ALARA principle, achieving sufficient image quality to assess lung density accurately but no higher, with the effective dose range between 1 and 10 mSv. The 20 mAs study had an effective dose of 0.7 mSv. Phantom studies should be conducted to verify that the kV and mAs for the study would provide sufficient image quality for the chosen quantitative CT metric and keep the effective dose no higher than 10 mSv.

Scan Mode and Pitch

The optimal scan mode was spiral CT scanning, not axial scanning. The pitch settings were discussed and pitch values between 1.0 and 2.0 were acceptable. Pitch values greater than 2.0 were not acceptable because of adverse effects on image quality. Pitch values less than 1.0 increased radiation dose and were not recommended.

Detector Width and Recommended Axial Image Thickness and Spacing

The workshop recommended using an effective detector element z axis thickness of 1 to 1.25 mm, with the ability to reconstruct thin 1- to 1.25-mm axial images and thicker axial images with a slice thickness equal to or greater than 7 mm. The thinner slice thickness would be able to detect small foci of emphysema with greater image noise, and the thicker slices would have less noise but would also average out small foci of emphysema that were much smaller than 7 mm. The 16-row MDCT scanners would be able to accomplish this with scan times less than 12 seconds. The focus of the workshop was on determining abnormally low attenuating areas of lung density (see Chapter 5) as a measure of pulmonary emphysema. At the time of this workshop, the assessment of airway geometry, which requires slice thicknesses less than 1.5 mm, and submillimeter is better, was not a consideration. It was recognized that if lung texture was to be assessed, then the detector element thickness would need to be 1.25 mm or less.[4]

Image Reconstruction

At the time of this workshop, filtered back projection (FBP) was the only reconstruction method available for image reconstruction. Iterative reconstruction (IR) was still in the future for commercial clinical x-ray CT scanners. However, it was recognized that the reconstruction kernel used in FBP image reconstruction was very important in determining both image noise and image spatial resolution. It was recommended that a neutral kernel be used, which at the time for the GE CT scanners was the "Standard" FBP reconstruction kernel. This neutral kernel would not edge enhance or smooth the image. It is interesting to note that this recommendation for using a neutral kernel in FBP is still favored in the early 2020s for lung CT AI.[7]

Optimal Lung Volume—Total Lung Capacity (TLC)

There are two main issues related to lung volume and the scanning of the patient for the assessment of lung disease: lung volume and coaching versus spirometric gating. It was generally agreed that for the assessment of emphysema the recommended lung volume is TLC. It was recommended that careful coaching of the patient to TLC by the x-ray CT technologist was the best approach. The use of spirometric gating was not recommended, as it did not add sufficient value over careful coaching of the patient to a given lung volume (e.g., TLC, RV). It should be noted that careful coaching is the approach in patients who undergo pulmonary physiology testing to assess airflow and lung volumes.

Administration of Intravenous Iodinated X-ray CT Contrast Media

The administration of intravenous iodinated contrast material will increase the x-ray CT measures of lung density due to the photoelectric absorption of x-ray photons by the iodine atoms in the contrast material. The presence of the iodinated contrast in both the intravascular and extravascular extracellular compartments of the lung tissue increases the x-ray CT measures of lung tissue density in HU due to the presence of the iodine atoms, and not due to any real change in the lung tissue density in the absence of the contrast material. So it was recommended that the use of iodinated contrast material should not be used in studies to assess pulmonary emphysema using lung density measurements from x-ray CT.[7]

X-ray CT Phantoms for Image Quality Assessments

It was recommended that air calibration CT scans and CT scans of water phantoms should be used to calibrate the CT scanners daily to maintain the accuracy of the CT HU numbers. Anthropomorphic x-ray CT phantoms can also be used to assess the accuracy of the CT scanners assessments of the density of normal and emphysematous lung tissue. The use of dedicated x-ray lung CT phantoms is important in assessing CT scanner performance and maintaining CT image quality.[5,7]

CT Image Analysis

The 15th percentile was the quantitative CT metric recommended by this workshop to assess changes in lung density due to pulmonary emphysema (see Chapter 5).

Image Data Transfer, Analysis, and Storage

It was recommended that both the reconstructed lung CT images and the unreconstructed projection data be transferred to a central image analysis facility using either DVD media or direct image transfer over the internet. The unreconstructed projection data are very large files, much larger than the reconstructed CT images; are difficult to obtain from many commercial CT scanner manufacturers; and present difficult challenges for transfer using DVDs or direct internet transfer. However, having the projection data to reconstruct additional CT images with different kernels would provide the opportunity to apply advances in CT image reconstruction in the future and could improve CT image quality throughout a particular study cohort.

Summary of the Recommended Quantitative Lung CT Scanning Protocol

In summary, the 2001 "Workshop: Quantitative Computed Tomography Scanning in Longitudinal Studies of Emphysema" recommended the following parameters for the quantitative lung CT scanning protocol to assess emphysema: 16-row MDCT scanner, same manufacturer and model for each patient over the course of the study; x-ray tube peak voltage of 120 kV, x-ray tube current time product of 20 to 100 mAs; effective radiation dose between 0.7 and 10 mSv, spiral scan mode, pitch between 1.0 to 2.0, maximum detector element z-axis width of 1.25 mm; coach patient to TLC; FBP method of image reconstruction using a neutral kernel, such as the GE Standard CT kernel; DFOV to include just the lungs, reconstruct axial images with 1- to 1.25-mm thickness and 7-mm or greater slice thickness; no intravenous contrast media; quality control should include regular scanning of appropriate CT phantoms, projection data and reconstructed images should be saved, and transfer of image data to central image processing facility for research studies via the internet or on DVDs (Box 3.2).

BOX 3.2 ■ The 2001 "Workshop: Quantitative Computed Tomography Scanning in Longitudinal Studies of Emphysema" Recommended CT Scanning Protocol

1. MDCT scanner, 16-row or greater (see *Single versus Multiple Detector Row CT Scanners* in this chapter)
2. Use the same CT scanner manufacturer and model for the same patient over the course of a study
3. Effective radiation dose = 0.7–10 mSv
4. X-ray tube peak voltage = 120 kV
5. X-ray tube current time product = 20–100 mAs
6. Spiral scanning mode
7. Pitch = 1.0–2.0
8. Verbally coach patient to total lung capacity (TLC)
9. Display field of view (DFOV) just large enough to include both lungs——using a reconstruction matrix size of 512 × 512
10. Reconstruction method
    a. Filtered back projection (FBP)
    b. Neutral reconstruction kernel (e.g., no smoothing or edge enhancement)
11. Axial CT image slice width = 1.0–1.25 mm OR ≥7 mm
12. No intravenous contrast material
13. Regular quality control checks to include CT phantoms (see *X-ray CT Phantoms for Image Quality Assessments* in this chapter)
14. CT projection data along with reconstructed CT images should be transmitted to a central image processing facility using the internet or on DVDs

Current Recommended Quantitative CT Scanning Protocol

The current recommendations for quantitative CT (QCT) scanning protocols to support lung CT AI work were described in a more recent publication entitled: "SPIROMICS Protocol for Multicenter Quantitative Computed Tomography to Phenotype the Lungs."[7] This study built on previous studies that helped develop QCT scanning protocols, including the 2001 workshop previously discussed.[3–5] This paper details a holistic approach that is described as the QCT lung assessment system (QCT-LAS). The QCT-LAS includes QCT imaging protocols for specific models of CT scanners for the assessment of lung disease at two lung volumes, TLC and RV. QCT-LAS includes monthly scanning of a standardized lung-specific CT phantom, in addition to scanning more traditional CT quality control phantoms. QCT-LAS includes web-based tools for patient/subject registration, CT protocol assignment, internet image data transmission, and automated CT image assessment to ensure that the proper CT scanning protocol was followed.[7]

RADIATION DOSE

The SPIROMICS CT Imaging Protocol uses the same x-ray tube peak voltage of 120 kV for all CT scanners but adjusts the x-ray tube current time product (mAs) to ensure that each CT scanner model outputs the same $CTDI_{vol}$ radiation dose. This standardizes the radiation exposure to subjects/patients when different CT scanner models are used.[7] As discussed in Chapter 2, the use of x-ray tube peak voltage modulation is not used in QCT applications due to the change in x-ray beam energy spectrum that occurs in this dose reducing scheme. There is a need to tailor the $CTDI_{vol}$ dose to the patient and, rather than use either x-ray tube peak voltage or x-ray tube current modulation, the SPIROMICS CT Imaging Protocol adjusts the tube current so that a smaller patient receives a smaller dose and a larger patient receives a larger dose. This is summarized in Table 3.1.[7] For example, the TLC CT scan for a small patient, BMI < 20, will use a $CTDI_{vol}$ of 6.1 mGy. The TLC CT scan for a medium patient, BMI between 20 and 30, will use a $CTDI_{vol}$ of 7.6 mGy. The TLC CT scan for a large patient, BMI > 30, will use a $CTDI_{vol}$ of 11.4 mGy.[7] The RV doses are less than the TLC doses since lung density measurements are derived from the RV scans and not any measurements of the airway or vessel structures. This has been shown to work well in the SPIROMICS study.[7]

MDCT SCANNER MODELS, SCAN MODE, Z-AXIS DETECTOR SIZE, ROTATION TIME, PITCH

The SPIROMICS CT Imaging Protocol specifies the number of z-axis detector channels, the z-axis detector width, and x-ray tube rotation time and pitch to try to harmonize the acquisition of image data coming from different CT vendors and CT models.[7] The use of an MDCT scanner with 64 rows/channels or more is recommended. These MDCT scanners need to have an effective z-axis detector element width of less than 1 mm and are typically in the range of 0.625 to 0.75 mm. Spiral scanning mode

TABLE 3.1 ■ **Computed Tomography Radiation Standardization**

Scan Type	Body Habitus	BMI Range	CTDI$_{vol}$ (mGy)
Inspiration	Obese	>30	11.4
Inspiration	Normal	20–30	7.6
Inspiration	Below normal	<20	6.1
Expiration	Obese	>30	6.1
Expiration	Normal	<30	4.2
Expiration	Below normal	<30	4.2

CT dose is standardized so each manufacturer and model is matched within ±3% of the target CTDI$_{vol}$. Adjustments to delivered dose were made on the basis of BMI ranges. Expiration radiation exposure uses the same CTDI$_{vol}$ for both normal and below-normal body sizes.
BMI = body mass index; CT = computed tomography; CTDI$_{vol}$ = volumetric computed tomography dose index.
Reprinted with permission of the American Thoracic Society. Copyright © 2022 American Thoracic Society. All rights reserved. (Table 3.1 from Sieren JP, Newell JD Jr., Barr RG, Bleecker ER, Burnette N, Carretta EE, et al. SPIROMICS protocol for multicenter quantitative computed tomography to phenotype the lungs. *Am J Respir Crit Care Med*. 2016;194(7):794–806). The American Journal of Respiratory and Critical Care Medicine is an official journal of the American Thoracic Society.

is recommended with an x-ray tube rotation time of 0.5 seconds and a pitch between 0.923 and 1.0. The scan times for a large thorax, 30 cm in z-axis length, are less than 10 seconds.

DFOV, ISOCENTER, SCANNING AT TLC AND RV

The SPIROMICS CT scanning protocol emphasizes the importance of scanning at a DFOV for the TLC CT scan that includes the lungs, and as little of the chest wall as possible, to maximize the in-plane resolution using a 512 × 512 reconstruction matrix (see Chapter 2). The same DFOV is used for both the TLC and RV scans to maintain the same in-plane resolution between the CT scans obtained at different lung volumes. The protocol is very specific in making sure the patient is scanned at the isocenter of the CT scanner, which minimizes cone beam and scatter artifacts in the reconstructed images. The protocol indicates that the arms of the patient should be above their heads but well supported and relaxed. There are very specific instructions for how the CT technologist should verbally coach the patient to the proper lung volume, TLC vs RV, and not use computer-generated voice commands.

CT IMAGE RECONSTRUCTION

FBP is used to reconstruct the CT images using a neutral kernel, such as the GE Standard CT kernel. The images are reconstructed with a thickness between 0.625 mm and 0.75 mm, and an interval between images of 0.5 mm, to achieve a nearly isotropic voxel size across multiple CT scanner models. Additional image reconstructions can be done if needed to achieve additional goals of a clinical or research CT study, including optimal reconstructions for visual CT assessment of lung disease.

QUALITY CONTROL

There are multiple issues that are addressed in the SPIROMICS CT scanning protocol regarding CT scanner calibration, CT image quality, and CT image data transfer. These have been incorporated into the QCT-LAS system.[7] The QCT-LAS system was designed for multicenter research studies of lung disease, such as SPIROMICS that need CT scans of the lungs. This system uses a web-based computer program that automates most of the steps, from authorizing the scan to confirming the CT image data received by the central processing facility meets study QC requirements, or indicating what QC issues need to be addressed.

Personnel Training and Certification

Study coordinators and CT technologists receive study-specific training. Upon the completion of training, they receive a unique identifier (ID) and password (PW) so they can log on to the QCT-LAS web-based software system. The ID and PW can be suspended, if needed, and remedial training done before the ID and PW are re-issued.

CT Scanner Calibration and Certification

Each CT scanner must complete two levels of initial certification.[7] The first level of CT scanner certification is met by scanning the manufacturer's CT model-specific CT phantom or suitable alternative (e.g., ACR CT phantom), to ensure the CT scanner is performing properly (meeting specific spatial and contrast resolution specifications, and ensuring that the HU numbers for standardized CT materials are accurate, e.g., air, water, acrylic). The second level of certification is having the CT scanner scan the COPDGene 1 phantom (see below under the heading *COPDGene CT Phantom*), which has very specific objects within the phantom that determine whether or not the scanner is able to assess the density of normal and abnormal lung tissue, and assess the size of airway lumens and airway walls.[10] The results from scanning the two phantoms are then entered into the QCT-LAS system for the specific CT scanner, and the system indicates if the scanner passed the level one and two certifications. Repeat scans of the two phantoms are performed at regular intervals (i.e., monthly), and these results are tracked in the QCT-LAS system to ensure these scans are not drifting over time. A 3 HU change in the density of one or more of the phantom materials scanned will cue alerts to indicate there is a potential problem with the CT scanner and corrective action must be taken before continuing use.

CT Scan Acquisition

The first step in using QCT-LAS to scan a subject/patient is for the study coordinator, or other authorized user, to log into the procedural verification software (PVS). The person logging into PVS must have a valid ID and PW for PVS. PVS checks to ensure that this is a certified user who has completed the necessary training to use the system. The study ID is then entered into PVS, and PVS finds an approved CT scanner at the study site that is up to date on all the necessary QC items. PVS checks the QCT-LAS database to find the BMI of the subject/patient and uses this information to print out the scan parameters to be used along with detailed instructions for the CT technologist, including positioning of the patient at isocenter; how to coach the patient to the proper lung volume (TLC or RV); selecting the proper DFOV; and ensuring the z-axis length of the scan is just long enough to include both lungs (minimizes the radiation dose to the subject/patient). PVS will check if the patient has had a previous CT for a particular study, and ensure the subject/patient is scanned on the same CT scanner and the same CT scan parameters are used.

CT Image Data Transfer

The next step is for the study coordinator, or other authorized person, to log into DICOM Selection Parser and Transfer Check (DISPATCH) software. This is an automated system that imports the CT scan data at the clinical center and exports the data over the internet to the offsite CT image data center.[7] DISPATCH checks the CT DICOM header for the set of CT images that were obtained to ensure that proper CT scanning parameters were selected. It also checks the volume of the lungs in the TLC and RV scans. If the CT study passes all of the checks, the study coordinator is notified that the data is accepted. If DISPATCH detects problems with the CT study, email notifications are sent to the study site and the offsite CT image data center so that any correctable quality issues can be addressed before the unreconstructed projection data residing on the CT scanner is deleted. Correctable CT scanning protocol errors include incorrect DFOV, reconstruction kernel, slice thickness, or slice interval. These errors can be avoided by using this near real-time notification feature of DISPATCH. Uncorrectable CT image quality issues generate emails to various authorized study personnel that describe the shortcomings of the CT study. Uncorrectable CT study errors include improper patient positioning, motion artifacts, improper radiation dose, and improper lung volumes. DISPATCH also keeps track of the errors that occur, and provides QC reports for the different study sites and CT technologists. These QC reports are reviewed, and corrective action taken to address CT scanner calibration issues and CT technologist remedial training. Box 3.3 summarizes the SPIROMICS CT Scanning Protocol.

CT Scanner Quality Control
CT SCANNER QUALITY CONTROL MEASURES, ACR CT PHANTOM

Visual and quantitative CT scanning protocols need a CT scanner quality control program that include procedures performed on a daily, monthly, and annual basis, as described in the American College of Radiology's 2017 Computed Tomography Quality Control Manual.[11] On a daily basis, the CT technologist warms up the x-ray tube, performs air calibrations, and scans a CT water phantom. The CT technologist will first warm up the x-ray tube. Then, the CT technologist will follow the manufacturer's procedures for performing an air calibration of the CT scanner. The air calibration is completed by performing a CT scan with nothing in the gantry to assess how the different x-ray detector elements record essentially the same information, the density of air. Then, both spiral and axial mode CT scans are performed using either the scanner manufacturer's water phantom or the ACR's CT phantom to assess the mean and standard deviation in HUs of water and assess for any artifacts.[11,12] The average HU value of water should be 0 ± 3 HU, and the value must be within 0 ± 5 HU when using the

---

BOX 3.3 ■ 2016 SPIROMICS Protocol for MDCT to Phenotype the Lungs

1. 64-row or greater MDCT scanner
2. Use the same CT scanner for the same patient over the course of a study
3. Absorbed radiation dose = see Table 3.1 (ALARA)
4. X-ray tube peak voltage = 120 kV (no kV modulation)
5. X-ray tube current time product = see Table 3.1 (no tube current modulation)
6. Spiral scanning mode
7. X-ray tube rotation time = 0.5 seconds
8. Scan time for 30 cm scan length <10 seconds
9. Pitch = 0.923–1.0 (use pitch length value 1.0 or as close as possible)
10. Verbally coach patient to total lung capacity (TLC) or residual volume (RV)
11. Display field of view (DFOV) just large enough to include both lungs—using a reconstruction matrix size of 512 × 512
12. Reconstruction method
    a. Filtered back project (FBP)
    b. Neutral reconstruction kernel (e.g., no smoothing or edge enhancement)
13. Axial CT image slice width = 0.625–0.75 mm (use minimum slice width available)
14. Axial CT slice interval = 0.5 mm
15. No intravenous contrast material
16. Regular quality control checks to include CT phantoms (see *X-ray CT Phantoms for Image Quality Assessments* in this chapter)
17. CT projection data along with reconstructed CT images should be transmitted to a central image processing facility using the internet (see *Image Data Transfer, Analysis, and Storage* in this chapter)

---

manufacturer's water phantom. The average value of water should be 0 ± 5 HU and within 0 ± 7 HU when using the ACR phantom.[11] The CT technologist will verify that all of the CT scanner controls and the gray level performance of the CT scanner computer display monitors are functioning properly on a monthly basis.[11] The CT medical physicist will perform the following quality control procedures on an annual basis: scout projection image prescription and alignment light accuracy, CT table travel accuracy, accuracy of the x-ray tube beam width, low-contrast accuracy of CT images, adequate spatial resolution of CT images, assess for any CT image artifacts, assess the accuracy of CT numbers, assess CT number uniformity, assess the radiation dose the CT scanner is producing, and assess the calibration of the CT scanner computer display monitors.[11] Spatial resolution and CT number accuracy can be assessed using the ACR phantom.[11] The spatial resolution for a neutral or standard kernel used for soft tissue assessments in the mediastinum and abdomen should be 6 LP/mm. The spatial resolution should increase to 8 LP/mm, using a sharp or edge enhancement kernel, for high-resolution CT (HRCT) of the lung.[11] The range of CT numbers for water should be 0 ± 7 HU, using an x-ray tube kilovoltage of 120 kV; −1000 HU is the CT number of air and the range should be between −970 HU and −1005 HU, using an x-ray tube peak voltage of 120 kV. It is important to scan using the 120 kV because, as discussed in Chapter 2, changing the x-ray tube peak kV will change the x-ray beam energy spectrum and the measured HU values of tissues.

COPDGENE CT PHANTOM

The Genetic Epidemiology of COPD (COPDGene) is a multicenter observational study that has been funded by NIH for over 10 years. COPDGene is designed to identify the genetic risk factors of developing COPD and the chest CT phenotypes of patients with COPD.[13] There are many different CT scanner models in this study with different CT manufacturers. The COPDGene 1 phantom is a custom-designed CT phantom developed to provide increased rigor in the quality control process for the multiple different CT scanner models in this study.[10]

The COPDGene phantom 1 is an oval shaped object that mimics the cross-sectional area of the thorax. It measures 350 mm × 250 mm × 50 mm[10] and contains a 250 mm × 150 mm oval insert made of "lung" equivalent foam (−856 HU). It also contains an 80 mm diameter acrylic cylinder (120 HU), 80 mm air-filled hole (−1000 HU), and 80 mm diameter cylindrical water containing bottle (0 HU). The COPDGene phantom also contains six polycarbonate tubes of varying sizes and thicknesses, which are used to assess how well the CT scanner determines the wall area and luminal area of the lung airways. CT scanning of the COPDGene phantom is an additional quality control procedure that has proven helpful in assessing and monitoring CT scanner performance over time, when multiple different CT scanner models from different manufacturers are used in a study. The COPDGene phantom can monitor the performance of many different CT scanners in determining the density of air, of lung equivalent foam, of water, and acrylic.[10]

Current QIBA Lung Density CT Profile

The Quantitative Imaging Biomarker Alliance (QIBA) of the Radiology Society of North America (RSNA) was founded in 2007, and its mission is to "improve the value and practicality of quantitative imaging biomarkers by reducing variability across devices, sites, patients, and time."[14] QIBA has developed imaging profiles that give specific guidelines on how best to acquire specific imaging biomarkers. There are coordinating committees for x-ray CT, MRI, Ultrasound, and Nuclear Medicine. Currently, the QIBA CT coordinating committee has three CT scanning profiles that are relevant to this book: QIBA CT Lung Density Profile, QIBA CT Tumor Volume Change for Advanced Disease Profile (nodules/masses greater than 10 mm in the lung), and the CT Small Lung Nodule Assessment and Monitoring in Low Dose Screening Profile (6 to 10 mm diameter lung nodules).[14]

The recommendations in the QIBA CT Lung Density Profile (QCTLDP) specify that to accurately determine the number of lung voxels less than −950 HU or the HU value of the 15th percentile of the lung voxel histogram curve (see Chapter 4), a 16-row or greater MDCT scanner should be utilized, using a $CTDI_{vol}$ of 3 mGy or less for an average size patient (75 kg).[15] The total scan time should be 10 seconds or less. If multiple time points are to be scanned on the same patient, then the same CT scanner make, model, and CT scanning protocol should be used for each time point. The CT detector array should be capable of generating contiguous images of 1.0 mm slice thickness, or less, of the whole lungs in a single breath-hold.[14] The full width half maximum (FWHM) of the line spread function for both in-plane and through-plane resolution should be 1.0 mm or less. The density of air within a CT scan of a CT phantom, the COPDGene 1 phantom, should be −1000 HU ± 6 HU and 0 HU ± 6 HU for water. The stability of the HU measurements should be established for the CT scanner by scanning a suitable CT phantom five times and confirming that the standard deviation of the mean value of air, lung equivalent foam, and water are 1 HU or less. The reconstruction method should be FBP and the reconstruction kernel should match the characteristics of the GE Standard FBP kernel. IR is not recommended at this time. Tube current modulation can be used. The patient should be positioned properly in the CT scanner gantry at the isocenter of the CT gantry. The patient needs to be properly coached to TLC by a properly trained CT technologist. The DFOV needs to be no greater than 2 cm outside the maximum extent of the lung. No intravenous or oral contrast medium should be used. The length of the CT scan of the thorax should be no greater than 2 cm above the cranial portion of the lungs and no greater than 5 cm caudal to the lungs. The x-ray tube peak kilovoltage is not specifically mentioned, but 120 kV is implied based on the example references.[15] The QIBA Lung Density CT Protocol are summarized in Box 3.4.

Summary

The development of x-ray CT scanning protocols for QCT and lung CT AI has been developed over several decades and continues to be an active area of research and development. MDCT scanners with 64 rows or more are preferred in lung QCT. These scanners provide short scanning times so even the most severely diseased lungs can be scanned in a single breath-hold. There is agreement that lung QCT scanning protocols should conform to the ALARA standard, and use only as much ionizing radiation as is necessary to achieve the most benefit and least risk for the patient. The length of the CT scan in the cranial caudal axis should be as short as possible to minimize the radiation dose to the patient. The tube current time product (mAs) should be tailored to the size of the patient, and this can be done by tube current modulation or selecting fixed mA values based on patient size, BMI. The x-ray tube peak kV should be set to a fixed value for a given study, for example 120 kV. X-ray tube peak voltage modulation is not recommended. The CT dose for an average 75-kg patient can be 3 mGy or less in many instances. Intravenous and oral contrast material should not be administered. The patient should be carefully placed at the isocenter of the CT gantry. The patient should be coached to the proper lung volume, TLC and/or RV, for the CT scan by a CT technologist trained in this procedure. The DFOV should include as little of the chest wall as

---

BOX 3.4 ■ 2020 QIBA Lung Density CT Protocol

1. MDCT scanner, 16-row or greater
2. Use the same CT scanner make and model for the same patient over the course of a study
3. Effective radiation dose = 3 mGy or less for 75 kg patient (ALARA)
4. X-ray tube peak voltage = 120 kV (no kV modulation)
5. X-ray tube current time product (mAs) is chose so radiation dose is 3 mGy or less (tube current modulation is permitted)
6. Spiral scanning mode
7. X-ray tube rotation time = 0.5 seconds
8. Scan time <10 seconds
9. Resolution—in-plane and through-plane resolution of 1 mm or less
10. Verbally coach patient in the supine position to total lung capacity (TLC)
11. Display field of view (DFOV) just large enough to include both lungs
    a. No more than 2 cm of tissue outside the lungs
    b. Reconstruction matrix size of 512 × 512
    c. Confirm patient is within 2 cm of isocenter
    d. Scan length from no greater than 2 cm above the lung apices to no lower than 5 cm below the lung bases
12. Reconstruction method
    a. Filtered back projection (FBP)
    b. Neutral reconstruction kernel (e.g., no smoothing or edge enhancement)
13. Axial CT image slice width = 1.0 mm or less
14. Axial CT slice interval = contiguous
15. No intravenous or oral contrast material
16. Extensive initial and regular quality control checks to include CT phantoms (see *X-ray CT Phantoms for Image Quality Assessments* in this chapter)
17. Reconstructed CT images should be transmitted in uncompressed DICOM format according to the anonymization standards for the approved study

---

(Adapted from RSNA. QIBA Profile: Computed Tomography: Lung Densitometry 2021. Accessed April 21, 2022. https://qibawiki.rsna.org/images/a/a8/QIBA_CT_Lung_Density_Profile_090420-clean.pdf.])

---

possible and still capture all of the lung; the same DFOV should be used on subsequent scans if the goals of the CT study have not changed.

The preferred image reconstruction method is FBP with a CT kernel performance similar to the GE Standard CT kernel. IR is used routinely in visual lung CT applications to reduce dose and/or image noise, and further research will hopefully provide IR methods that can be applied to QCT.

The CT image thickness should be 1 mm or less. The in-plane and through-plane CT image resolution should be 1 mm or less. The density of air should be −1000 HU ± 6 HU and 0 HU ± 6 HU for water. CT phantoms are very important in assessing the spatial and density resolution of CT scanners.

Automated real-time or near real-time monitoring of CT scan quality, and internet transfer of DICOM CT image data, is very helpful in correcting CT scanning errors that can be addressed by reconstructing the projection data stored on the CT scanner; for monitoring uncorrectable CT scanning errors; and for providing feedback to CT technologist and other healthcare or research personnel.

References

1. AAPM. Adult Routine Chest CT Protocols Version 2.1. 2016. Accessed April 9, 2020. https://www.aapm.org/pubs/CTProtocols/documents/AdultRoutineChestCT.pdf.
2. AAPM. Lung Cancer Screening CT Protocols Version 5.1. 2019. Accessed April 21, 2022. https://www.aapm.org/pubs/ctprotocols/documents/lungcancerscreeningct.pdf.
3. Newell Jr JD. Quantitative computed tomography of lung parenchyma in chronic obstructive pulmonary disease: an overview. *Proc Am Thorac Soc.* 2008;5(9):915–918.
4. Newell Jr JD, Hogg JC, Snider GL. Report of a workshop: quantitative computed tomography scanning in longitudinal studies of emphysema. *Eur Respir J.* 2004;23(5):769–775.
5. Newell Jr JD, Sieren J, Hoffman EA. Development of quantitative computed tomography lung protocols. *J Thorac Imaging.* 2013;28(5):266–271.
6. Newell Jr JD, Tschirren J, Peterson S, Beinlich M, Sieren J. Quantitative CT of interstitial lung disease. *Semin Roentgenol.* 2019;54(1):73–79.
7. Sieren JP, Newell Jr. JD, Barr RG, Bleecker ER, Burnette N, Carretta EE, et al. SPIROMICS protocol for multicenter quantitative computed tomography to phenotype the lungs. *Am J Respir Crit Care Med.* 2016;194(7):794–806.
8. Dirksen A, Dijkman JH, Madsen F, Stoel B, Hutchison DC, Ulrik CS, et al. A randomized clinical trial of alpha(1)-antitrypsin augmentation therapy. *Am J Respir Crit Care Med.* 1999;160(5 Pt 1):1468–1472.
9. NHLBI. The definition of emphysema. Report of a National Heart, Lung, and Blood Institute, Division of Lung Diseases workshop. *Am Rev Respir Dis.* 1985;132(1):182–185.
10. Sieren JP, Newell JD, Judy PF, Lynch DA, Chan KS, Guo J, et al. Reference standard and statistical model for intersite and temporal comparisons of CT attenuation in a multicenter quantitative lung study. *Med Phys.* 2012;39(9):5757–5767.
11. Dillon C, Breeden W, Clements J, Cody D, Gress D, Kanal K, et al. 2017 Computed Tomography Quality Control Manual. Accessed April 21, 2022. https://www.acr.org/-/media/ACR/Files/Clinical-Resources/QC-Manuals/CT_QCManual.pdf.
12. McCollough CH, Bruesewitz MR, McNitt-Gray MF, Bush K, Ruckdeschel T, Payne JT, et al. The phantom portion of the American College of Radiology (ACR) computed tomography (CT) accreditation program: practical tips, artifact examples, and pitfalls to avoid. *Med Phys.* 2004;31(9):2423–2442.
13. Regan EA, Hokanson JE, Murphy JR, Make B, Lynch DA, Beaty TH, et al. Genetic epidemiology of COPD (COPDGene) study design. *COPD.* 2010;7(1):32–43.
14. RSNA. Quantitative Imaging Biomarker Alliance: RSNA. Updated 7 March 2022. Accessed April 21, 2022. https://qibawiki.rsna.org/index.php/Profiles.
15. RSNA. QIBA Profile: Computed Tomography: Lung Densitometry 2021. Accessed April 4, 2022. https://qibawiki.rsna.org/images/a/a8/QIBA_CT_Lung_Density_Profile_090420-clean.pdf.

Quantitative Assessment of Lung Nodule Size, Shape, and Malignant Potential Using Both Reactive and Limited-Memory Lung CT AI

CT Assessment of Lung Nodules—CT Versus Projection Radiography (PR)

This chapter will describe the importance of detecting and assessing the risk of lung cancer in a lung nodule by lung CT AI. The diameter of the pulmonary nodule was the first widely used research and clinical quantitative CT (QCT) metric derived from chest CT scans and predated the use of clinical QCT metrics of diffuse lung disease by several decades.[1] This chapter introduces the topic of the solitary pulmonary nodule and the importance of assessing these nodules using multiple QCT metrics that help in determining the malignant potential of a lung nodule.

A lung nodule is a spherical structure of soft tissue density, approximately 40 HU, replacing the normal lung tissue with a diameter between 3 and 30 mm (Fig. 4.1).[2,3] The important features of a lung nodule include size, shape, density, contour, texture, and also assessing tissue features of the lung tissue adjacent to the lung nodule (Box 4.1).[3,4] It is very common to detect a nodule in screening populations that are at high risk for lung cancer.[3] At least one nodule is detected in up to 51% of these patients, and greater than 95% of these nodules are benign.[3] For this reason, there has been much research into determining what specific CT features of a lung nodule determine if it is benign or malignant. The size of the solitary pulmonary nodule is a simple feature that is a very strong predictor of the risk that the etiology of the nodule is due to lung cancer.[3]

The detection and assessment of pulmonary nodules were an early strength of x-ray CT due to the true 3D assessment of the lung anatomy and increased contrast resolution compared to 2D x-ray projection radiographic imaging.[1] The chest CT scan provides a 3D visualization of the lungs compared to the 2D representation that projection imaging generates, such as digital chest radiography. When a frontal and lateral 2D digital projection image of the chest is obtained on a person with suspected lung disease, the visual interpretation relies on the expert imaging physician being able to generate a 3D image of the lung anatomy in their brain, and this has its limitations. The chest CT is a more capable imaging method in the detection, localization, and assessment of nodule characteristics compared to projection radiography.[5] This is due to chest CT's accurate 3D depiction of the lung anatomy, high tissue contrast, compared to projection radiography, and the quantitative assessment of nodule features that are determined by the CT voxel size and HU value assigned to each voxel.

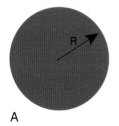

A

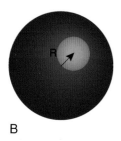

B

Fig. 4.1 Graphical descriptions of a spherical soft tissue lung nodule. The formulas for calculating the area and volume using the radius of the lung nodule are also shown. **(A)** 2D view of ideal spherical lung nodule; Area $= \pi \times R^2$. **(B)** 3D view of ideal spherical lung nodule; Volume $= 4/3 \times \pi \times R^3$.

BOX 4.1 ■ Important Imaging Features in Lung Nodules

- Shape
- Size
- Density in HU
- Contour
- Texture
- Adjacent lung parenchymal density and texture

There are multiple clinical situations where one or more lung nodules may be detected on chest CT scans. The etiology of the lung nodule is most commonly due to prior infection, current infection, lung cancer, or metastatic cancer. There are multiple clinical scenarios, each with important considerations in the assessment of lung nodule(s). We will focus on two of these clinical scenarios: incidental lung nodules detected on noncontrast chest CT scans, and lung nodules detected on noncontrast low-dose chest CT scans as part of an approved ACR lung cancer screening program for high-risk smokers.[6]

CT PROTOCOL TO ASSESS LUNG NODULES

Nodule detection and the assessment of nodule size, shape, contour, density, and texture are important because lung cancer commonly presents as a solitary lung nodule, and the size and other CT features of the nodule can help in determining if the nodule is cancer or due to a benign tumor or infection. The best treatment approach is to detect a cancerous lung nodule when it is small and have it removed before it has spread to other structures within and/or outside of the thorax. Accurately detecting and following the size and other important features of a lung nodule require adherence to recommended CT scanning protocols, CT scanner quality assurance, and routine use of CT scanner lung nodule phantoms or test objects.[7] A CT slice thickness of 2 mm or less is required to assess important features of the lung nodule.[8] The size of a lung nodule increases on expiration and decreases on inspiration, so consistent inspiratory effort is necessary for the initial assessment of lung nodules and to accurately follow the size of the lung nodule over time. It has been reported that the mean change in nodule volume increases 23% between inspiration and expiration.[3] The size, density, contour, and textural pattern of lung nodules are affected by slice thickness and reconstruction kernel. A neutral reconstruction kernel and narrow slice thickness represent the most accurate way of assessing lung nodule size, density, contour, and texture. A larger slice thickness (>2 mm) will reduce the size of the nodule due to partial volume effects at the surface of the nodule. The smaller the nodule, the greater this effect. The smooth kernel and large slice thickness (>2 mm) will average out important density, contour, and textural features. A sharp kernel will introduce artifacts within the nodule that will affect the accuracy of density and texture measurements. There are well-established quantitative criteria for the assessment of lung nodule size, growth, density, contour, and morphology.[7,9]

CT Determination of Lung Nodule Size

The size of a lung nodule is a powerful predictor of whether a lung nodule is benign or due to a malignant cancer. The larger the nodule size, the greater the risk of lung cancer (Fig. 4.2).[10–12] Multiple research studies have shown that the risk of lung cancer in a small lung nodule (<5 mm in diameter) is negligible, even in high-risk patients, or negligible for a new nodule.[3] The odds of a lung nodule being malignant increase between 1.1 and 1.15 times for every 1 mm increase in diameter above 4 mm.[3] The prevalence of malignancy in nodules equal to or greater than 20 mm is greater than 64%.[3] Currently, the QCT determination of lung nodule size is most commonly assessed by measuring

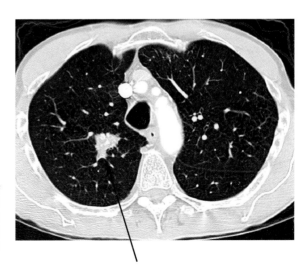

Fig. 4.2 Axial chest CT image of a 3-cm lobulated, spiculated solid soft tissue lung nodule *(arrow)* in the RUL that is suspicious for lung cancer in a patient with underlying emphysema from COPD.[10–12]

the diameter of the nodule, and this is most commonly performed by the expert imaging physician visually interpreting the chest CT scan. The recommended interactive quantitative method to determine the average diameter of a lung nodule that is less than 10 mm in diameter is first to determine the longest diameter of the nodule on an axial, coronal, or sagittal lung CT image and then use the same imaging plane to obtain the shortest one-dimensional diameter of the nodule.[10] Then the longest and shortest diameters of the nodule are used to calculate the average diameter of the nodule.[6] Accurate linear measurements of anatomic structures on chest CT images, including nodule diameters, can be done using the interactive AI measuring tools available in the picture archiving and communication system (PACS) software. PACS used by expert imaging physicians to quantitatively assess the size of lung nodules detected on chest CT scans. This is the method recommended in the American College of Radiology Lung Imaging Reporting and Data System, Lung-RADS.[3] There are AI agent software programs that can automatically calculate the diameter and volume of a lung nodule, but these AI agents require very specific CT scanning protocols to accurately determine the average diameter and volume of the lung nodule.[13] The size of a lung nodule can change by simply using a different AI software program; by using expiratory instead of an inspiratory CT scan; or by using a thicker slice thickness instead of a thin slice thickness, and between standard and reduced dose CT scanning protocols.[3] The volumetric approach is the best approach if the technical issues are all addressed properly.[3,13]

CT Determination of Nodule Growth

The growth of a solid soft tissue lung nodule on sequential chest CT scans indicates that this is an active lesion, and the two most common etiologies are active infection or cancer. A solid soft tissue lung nodule that remains stable in size for over 2 years is presumed to be benign. There are also ground-glass and part-solid type nodules.[6] A ground-glass nodule has increased density compared to a normal lung, but the normal lung vessels and outer airway wall can still be seen within the confines of the ground-glass nodule. The part-solid nodule has both ground-glass and solid soft tissue components. The solid soft tissue component obscures the normal lung vessels and the outer wall of airways. Ground-glass nodules and part-solid nodules equal to or greater than 6 mm need to be followed for a longer period of time, typically up to 5 years, to confirm they are benign.[6] The growth of the nodule can be determined by assessing the interval increase in the nodule's diameter, area, or volume. Lung CT AI software that assesses the volume of the nodule at multiple time points improves the accuracy of assessing nodule growth when compared to manual measurements of nodule diameter, area.[3]

The time it takes a nodule to double in volume, volume doubling time (VDT), is helpful in determining if a solid soft tissue lung nodule is benign or malignant. Most malignant solid soft tissue lung nodules have a VDT between 20 and 400 days. Most nonmalignant lung nodules will have a doubling time less than 20 days or more than 400 days.[3] The VDT of ground-glass nodules has been reported to be 628.5 days, and the VDT for part-solid nodules has been reported as 276.9 days.[3] It is important to recall from the above discussion on the assessment of lung nodule size that nodule volumetric software using specific CT scanning protocols will produce the best results in assessing the VDT of lung nodules over time, but the same software and rigorous CT scanning protocol need to be used at each time point.[3]

Milanese et al. (2018) reported the results of using the ClearRead lung CT AI nodule volume program (ClearRead CT, Riverain Technologies, Miamisburg, OH, USA) on nodules detected using chest CT.[14] The chest CT scan protocol used the Siemens SOMATOM Force third-generation dual-source MDCT scanner is 100 kVp with tin filtration, reference tube-current product of 45 mAs, pitch of 1.2, collimation 96 × 0.6 mm, and a gantry rotation time of 0.5 seconds. The reconstructed image matrix was the standard 512 × 512. The reconstructed images used a slice thickness of 2 mm, slice increment of 1.6 mm, and the B64 sharp reconstruction kernel with the advanced modeled iterative reconstruction (ADMIRE) strength of 3.[14] The ClearRead AI program removes the vessels from the lung CT images to enhance the detection and increase the accuracy of the nodule size measurements made interactively by expert imaging physicians, and by software programs designed to determine the volume of lung nodules seen on chest CT images. Nodules that are ill defined or adjacent to vessels are more difficult for AI nodule segmentation programs to characterize accurately. The standard chest CT images are referred to as SCT. The ClearRead processed lung CT images, which have the vessels and airways removed, are referred to as vessel suppressed CT (VSCT).[14] The study included 93 patients that ranged in age from 20 to 80 years with a median age of 56 years. There were 24 females and 59 males. Seventy-seven solid soft tissue nodules were detected in 43 of the 93 subjects. Semiautomated measurements of nodule volume were done on 77 nodules. Manual correction of nodule volume segmentation was necessary in 49 of the 77 nodules (75%). Twelve nodules were excluded from the analysis because their volume exceeded 400 mm³. The 65 remaining nodules varied in volume from 13 to 366 mm³.

Each SCT and VSCT set of images were transferred to a workstation that was also running a dedicated computer-aided nodule detection software program, MM Oncology. One radiologist and the MM Oncology software program were both used to identify the nodules on the SCT images. The MM Oncology program was also used to semiautomatically calculate nodule maximum diameter, corresponding maximum orthogonal diameter, and volume for the SCT dataset. The radiologist used a five-point scale to assess the likelihood that each of the nodules detected by either the radiologist viewing the SCT images or the MM Oncology software program processing the SCT images were, in fact, lung nodules. The nodule scores assigned by the radiologist were: (1) no nodule, (2) no confident nodule, (3) probable nodule, (4) more definite nodule, and (5) definite nodule. Those nodules with a score of 3 or more were included in the study. The radiologist also indicated the location of the nodule: subpleural, adjacent to fissures, within 2 cm of the pleura, and central nodules. Contact between the nodule and a pulmonary vessel was also noted. The spatial coordinates of the included nodules were also included to allow for the matching of nodules on the VSCT-processed images.

Then, the radiologist and a radiologist resident independently performed semiautomatic segmentations of the 65 solid soft tissue nodules in the study using both SCT with MM Oncology software and VSCT.[14] The volumes and longest diameters obtained using SCT and MM Oncology software by each reader were averaged, and these QCT metrics formed the reference standard to evaluate how well the ClearRead VSCT AI software performed.

The semiautomated volumetric lung nodule measurements on VSCT for the radiologist and the radiology resident showed substantial agreement when compared to the SCT/MM Oncology reference standard.[14] There was nearly perfect agreement for the volumetric assessment of central nodules and nodules adjacent to a pulmonary vessel between the two readers using VSCT, compared to SCT/MM Oncology. There was substantial agreement for the volumetric assessment between the two readers for peripheral nodules and subpleural/perifissural nodules, compared to the SCT/MM Oncology reference standard.[14] The longest diameter of each nodule showed substantial agreement between VSCT and SCT/MM Oncology for both the radiologist and the radiology resident.

The results of this study show that two independent methods of assessing nodule volume are in close agreement for both a radiologist and a radiology resident. The remaining challenge is to develop accurate, fully automatic segmentation of lung nodules to assess their volume and other desired size metrics over time, to help determine if the nodule is benign or malignant.

CT Determination of Nodule Density

The density of a soft tissue lung nodule is about 40 HU, which is similar to the CT density of muscle or solid organs.[3] The visual or quantitative density assessment of a lung nodule is most reliable when a neutral reconstruction kernel is used, the slice thickness needs to be equal to or less than 2.5 mm but a slice thickness of 1.0 mm or less is preferred, if possible.[8] The density features of a lung nodule can be assessed visually or quantitatively. The presence of visible fat in the lung nodule, Hounsfield number range −140 HU to −30 HU, indicates that the nodule is most likely a benign hamartoma or, rarely, a lipoma.[3] The presence of certain patterns of calcium in the lung nodule can indicate that it is not a malignant tumor but due to prior infection, or it is a benign tumor of the lung. Calcium has a CT density number greater than 175 HU.[3] There are four patterns of calcification that suggest the nodule is benign diffuse, central (<10% calcified), symmetric lamellar, and symmetric popcorn (Fig. 4.3). The first three patterns suggest the nodule is due to prior granulomatous disease infection of the lung, such as mycobacterium tuberculosis or fungal infection. The fourth configuration, popcorn, can be seen most commonly in patients with a benign hamartoma-type tumor of the lung. There are occasions when other patterns of calcification occur in a lung nodule, but these can be seen in both malignant tumors and benign causes of lung nodules.

There are three soft tissue nodule density patterns: solid, part-solid, and ground-glass (Fig. 4.4). The solid nodule, previously discussed in CT Determination of Nodule Growth, replaces the normal lung density airways and vessels and is typically about 40 HU in density.[2,3,15] The following discussion relates to full inspiratory chest CT scans, and chest CT scans obtained at total lung capacity (TLC). The ground-glass nodule has increased density compared to normal lung density, −846 HU, but is less dense than the solid nodule.[3,16] The walls of the airways and pulmonary vessels are still visible within the ground-glass nodule. The part-solid nodule has both solid and ground-glass density patterns.[2,3,6] The malignant rate of solid soft tissue nodules is 7%, ground-glass is nodules is 18%, and part-solid nodules is 63%.[3] The odds ratio for malignancy of a part-solid nodule greater than 6 mm in size, compared to a solid nodule of the same size, is 1.4.[3]

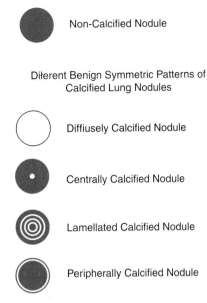

Non-Calcified Nodule

Diferent Benign Symmetric Patterns of Calcified Lung Nodules

Diffiusely Calcified Nodule

Centrally Calcified Nodule

Lamellated Calcified Nodule

Peripherally Calcified Nodule

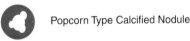

Popcorn Type Calcified Nodule

Fig. 4.3 Graphical description of the benign symmetric patterns of calcification in lung nodules on chest CT scans.

The odds ratio for malignancy of a ground-glass nodule, compared to a solid soft tissue nodule, is 0.8.[3]

The presence of air within a small nodule is helpful. Part-solid and ground-glass nodules with air bronchograms and small air-containing cysts are very suggestive of adenocarcinoma of the lung.[3] The presence of gas within a solid soft tissue nodule suggests active infection or a primary or secondary (metastatic) malignant tumor of the lung. The thickness of the wall of a cavity helps assess the etiology of cavitating solid soft tissue nodules. A wall thickness less than 4 mm suggests a benign etiology, usually infection. When the wall thickness is between 5 and 15 mm in diameter, there is a 50% chance the lesion is malignant. When the wall thickness is greater than 16 mm, it is very likely a malignant tumor.[3]

CT Determined Nodule Mass, Location, Morphology, Shape, Contour

The calculation of the mass, M, of a lung nodule can be determined from the mean attenuation of the nodule in HU, A_{mean}, and the volume, V, of the nodule using the following formula:

$$M = V \times (A_{mean} + 1000)$$

Nodule mass has been shown to decrease intraobserver and interobserver variation, compared to nodule volume calculations. Nodule mass calculations will likely be most useful in part-solid and ground-glass nodules.[3]

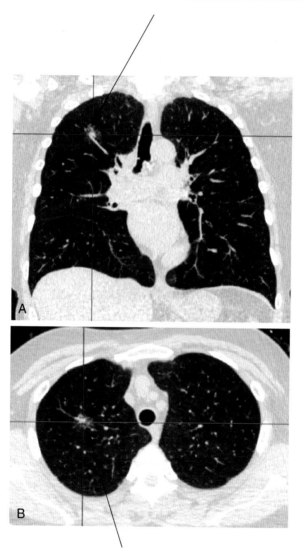

Fig. 4.4 Axial CT image **(A)** and coronal MPR CT image **(B)** of the chest with a part-solid soft tissue nodule due to adenocarcinoma *(arrows)* in the right upper lobe. Maximum diameter of the nodule is 22 mm and the maximum solid component diameter is 9 mm.

Lung cancer nodules are more likely to occur in the upper lobes.[3] The location of a solid soft tissue nodule with an elongated shape within 1.5 cm of a pulmonary fissure, or with a thin linear radiopaque opacity connecting the nodule to the pleural, makes it more likely that the nodule is benign and not malignant. These nodules are typically intrapulmonary lymph nodes.[3] A symmetrically round lung nodule is less likely to be malignant than a lobulated lung nodule. A lung nodule with an irregular, spiculated, or ill-defined contour is more likely to be a malignant nodule.[3]

CT Determined Nodule Texture—Limited-Memory AI

The above discussion relates to lung nodule features that are easily understood and assessed visually using expert imaging physicians and/or using reactive machine type AI software programs. Radiomics is an AI field that depends on reactive and limited-memory AI software programs to automatically assess quantitative imaging features from a set of medical images to derive features that cannot be derived by an expert imaging physician. Radiomics applied to the assessment of lung nodules detected on chest CT images assesses many QCT metrics of the lung nodule more precisely, and with greater capability, than the visual assessment of nodule size, density, and contour to determine if a given lung nodule's malignant potential. Wilson and Devaraj, in 2017, reviewed the application of radiomics to the assessment of the lung nodule.[17] In this review, the authors describe the ability of radiomics to determine histologic subtyping, gene expression, and prognosis following therapy of lung nodules.[17]

There are four steps in the lung CT AI assessment of lung nodules (Fig. 4.5). The first step is to use an appropriate CT scanning protocol to generate and display high-quality lung CT images to use in the AI evaluation of the lung nodule. This will be described in more detail below and builds on the information in Chapters 1 through 3.

The second step is to identify and segment the nodule(s), and in some instances the adjacent lung parenchyma, from the surrounding lung tissue.[4] Ideally, the lung nodule(s) are segmented automatically by the AI program so no manual editing is necessary. Currently, it is often necessary for the manual editing of AI-identified nodules; more robust AI tools to automatically segment the lung nodule is an ongoing area of research.

The third step in the radiomic AI analysis is to capture important features of the nodule. The radiomic AI program will capture features that have been previously discussed, and are easily understood in terms of visual inspection of the lung nodule, including volume and contour. As previously discussed, the assessment of nodule volume and doubling time are more precisely and accurately determined using AI software approaches than manual methods using electronic calipers. The next level of radiomic feature analysis of lung nodules is the assessment of the voxel histogram of the lung nodule, including assessment of the mean, variance, skewness, and kurtosis of the lung nodule voxel histogram. The next level is to use machine learning to assess texture features of the nodules, which looks at the relationship of voxel values in the neighborhood of a given voxel. An example of this is nodule entropy, which assesses the randomness of neighboring voxel values within the nodule.[17] Wavelet analysis has also been applied to nodule feature extraction to assess nodule texture and intensity.[17] Deep machine learning approaches would be the next AI level in classifying the nodules (see below).

The fourth step in the radiomics AI assessment of lung nodules is to take all of the features of the lung nodule and use statistical methods, or machine learning strategies, limited-memory AI, to train an AI algorithm on a given training set of chest CT studies to classify a lung nodule into different categories, such as benign nodule or malignant nodule.[17] The trained AI algorithm is then validated on a separate group of cases from the same cohort to see if the performance of the AI algorithm is robust. Then, the AI algorithm is typically tested on an independent set of cases to further test the robustness of the AI algorithm to classify the lung nodule into different categories, such as benign or malignant.

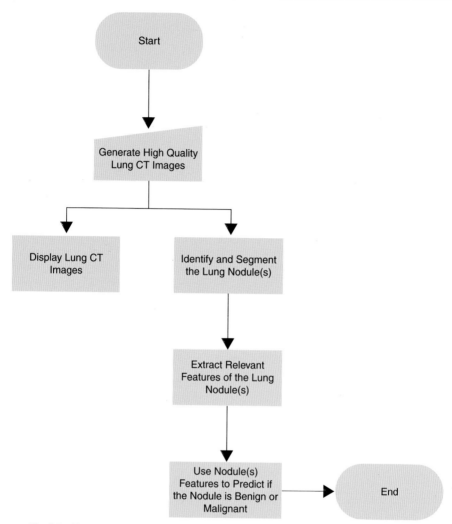

Fig. 4.5   Four steps that are essential in the lung CT AI assessment of lung nodules.

In one study looking at a radiomic approach to assess the malignant potential of solid soft tissue lung nodules, a large number of radiomic texture features were extracted and used to classify the lung nodules into either benign or malignant. There were 583 nodule features of intensity, shape, and heterogenicity used to classify 127 different indeterminant lung nodules into either a benign or malignant category. This study achieved an accuracy of 82.7% in classifying the lung nodule as benign or malignant.[17,18]

Radiomic texture features were used to assess whether 86 part-solid lung nodules, 31 transient nodules, and 47 persistent nodules, detected on chest CT in 77 individuals were transient nodules or persistent nodules.[17,19] This study showed that using the C statistic to assess the performance of the logistic regression analysis, when the clinical feature of blood eosinophilia and chest CT features of lesion size and multiplicity of lesions were used in the model, the AUC was 0.790. This study showed that the quantitative chest CT texture features of low mean attenuation, whole-nodule fifth percentile CT number, and higher positive skewness of CT attenuation determined from the voxel histogram of the nodule could be used to classify transient versus persistent part-solid lung nodules with an AUC of 0.831.[17,19] Combining blood eosinophilia, CT determined lesion size, and multiplicity with the above CT texture features, the AI classifier improved with the AUC increasing to 92.9%.[16,18]

Radiomics approaches to the assessment of lung nodules have resulted in a number of advances in assessing the malignant potential of a lung nodule; histological subtype of a given malignant lung nodule; expression of epidermal growth factor receptor (EGFR) mutations by malignant lung nodules; identifying K-ras mutations in malignant lung nodules; and assessing the response to different therapeutic approaches to the treatment of a malignant lung nodule.[17]

CT Assessment of Lung Tissue Adjacent to the Lung Nodule—Limited-Memory AI

There have been multiple successful reports using AI to assess whether lung nodules detected on chest CT were benign or malignant by assessing multiple QCT metrics of the lung nodule itself and also looking at multiple QCT metrics of the lung tissue adjacent to the lung nodule.[4]

Uthoff et al. (2019) reported the use of AI in assessing the malignant potential of lung nodules detected on chest CT scans using chest CT features derived from the lung nodule, and also from well-characterized zones of lung tissue adjacent to the lung nodule.[4] There were 363 lung nodules less than or equal to 30 mm in diameter retrospectively included in this study. There were 74 malignant nodules and 289 benign nodules in this cohort of 363 lung nodules that were used for the training of the AI algorithm. The subjects with lung nodules were obtained from three different well-characterized research studies: Genetic Epidemiology of Chronic Obstructive Lung Disease (COPDGene), National Lung Cancer Screening Trial (NLST), and the SPIE LungX Challenge.[4] The malignant nodules were all diagnosed using histopathology, and the benign nodules were diagnosed by either histopathology or longitudinal observation over 24 months demonstrating that the nodule was stable in size or had resolved. There were 100 lung nodules, 50 malignant and 50 benign, used for independent testing of the performance of the trained AI algorithm that was obtained from the INHALE study.[4]

Each of the lung nodules in the study was semiautomatically segmented into volumes of interest (VOI). Then four adjacent bands of lung tissue VOI were also semiautomatically segmented. The volumes of these four bands were determined by using 0.25, 0.50, 0.75, and 1.00 of the thickness of the nodule's largest in-plane diameter. The development of the AI algorithm included extracting QCT features from the nodule and the volume of each of the four parenchymal bands surrounding the nodule. These QCT features included 14 volumetric measures of the intensity histogram (V-IH), 136 volumetric Law's energy measures (V-LTEM), 13 volumetric gray-level run-length measures (V-GLRL), 13 volumetric gray-level size-zone measures (V-GLSZ), 5 volumetric neighborhood gray-tone difference measures (V-NGTD), and 17 measures of size and volumetric shape that included 11 border metrics (V-SzSp).[4] The QCT features were assessed for the nodule, 0.25 band, 0.50 band, 0.75 band, and 1.00 band. These five volumes were used to define a number of ANN networks.

The CT features of the lung nodule and the four surrounding tissue bands were further assessed by using the k-medoids machine learning method to generate k clusters with k representative medoid features.[4] The final set of features was determined using the information objective function maximum (IO_{max}). The selected features in each of the five volumes were used to train multiple artificial neural networks (ANN) with the performance of each ANN assessed through 10-fold cross-validation on a per-subject basis. Individual ANNs were initialized using random initialization of weights and then trained using stochastic gradient descent and hyperbolic tangent activation function.[4] The performance of each ANN network was assessed using the area under the curve for the receiver operating characteristic curve (AUC-ROC) and also the area under the precision-recall curve (AUC-PR).

The best-performing ANN tool included the nodule volume, 0.25 band volume, 0.50 band volume, and the 0.75 band volume. This is referred to as the Extended ML ANN. The Extended ML ANN included 50 features: 13 V-IH, 15 V-GLRL, 12 V-GLSZ, 6 V-NGTM, 1 B-ASC, and 3 V-SzSp. The performance of this Extended ML ANN, from the development cohort, achieved an AUC-ROC of 1.00 and an AUC-PR of 0.945. This represents perfect and near-perfect classification of benign and malignant nodules. The results of the Extended ML ANN on the independent validation cohort were AUC-ROC of 0.965 with an accuracy of 98%, sensitivity of 100%, and specificity of 96%.[4]

The high performance of the Extended ML ANN in correctly classifying benign from malignant nodules has great clinical significance. The Fleischner Society Pulmonary Nodule Follow-up Guidelines for the validation cohort that was derived from the INHALE study were compared to the management strategy of the Extended ML ANN. The Extended ML ANN identified 50 malignant nodules that would require Fleischner waiting periods between 3 and 12 months. The Extended ML tool identified 48 benign nodules that would have required a 3-month follow-up chest CT or biopsy. The application of the Extended ML ANN would have resulted in immediate treatment of malignant nodules without delay and would have eliminated any follow-up chest CT scans for the benign nodules in this study.[4]

The results of Uthoff's research show how limited-memory/machine learning AI software can increase the effectiveness of assessing whether a nodule on chest CT is benign or malignant compared to reactive machine AI algorithms that assess only the volume of a lung nodule. However, the results of limited-memory AI systems are very dependent on the data used to train and validate the AI algorithm.

The automatic and accurate segmentation of a lung nodule is an ongoing area of research and is a key technology enabler if advanced lung CT AI software programs using reactive machine or limited memory AI are to become widely used in research and clinical practice to automatically predict whether a lung nodule is benign or malignant, and to predict other important radiomic features of lung nodules as described in this chapter.

This chapter has introduced how lung CT AI can help assess important features of lung nodules and to help determine if a lung nodule is benign or malignant. The following chapter will look at how lung CT AI can be used to assess diffuse lung abnormalities, like emphysema, from COPD and pulmonary fibrosis from ILD.

References

1. Heitzman ER. Fleischner Lecture. Computed tomography of the thorax: current perspectives. *AJR Am J Roentgenol.* 1981;136(1):2–12.
2. Hansell DM, Bankier AA, MacMahon H, McLoud TC, Muller NL, Remy J. Fleischner Society: glossary of terms for thoracic imaging. *Radiology.* 2008;246(3):697–722.
3. Bartholmai BJ, Koo CW, Johnson GB, White DB, Raghunath SM, Rajagopalan S, et al. Pulmonary nodule characterization, including computer analysis and quantitative features. *J Thorac Imaging.* 2015;30(2):139–156.
4. Uthoff J, Stephens MJ, Newell Jr. JD, Hoffman EA, Larson J, Koehn N, et al. Machine learning approach for distinguishing malignant and benign lung nodules utilizing standardized perinodular parenchymal features from CT. *Med Phys.* 2019;46(7):3207–3216.
5. Aberle DR, Adams AM, Berg CD, Black WC, Clapp JD, et al. Reduced lung-cancer mortality with low-dose computed tomographic screening. National Lung Screening Trial Research (NLST). *N Engl J Med.* 2011;365(5):395–409.
6. MacMahon H, Naidich DP, Goo JM, Lee KS, Leung ANC, Mayo JR, et al. Guidelines for management of incidental pulmonary nodules detected on CT images: from the Fleischner Society 2017. *Radiology.* 2017;284(1):228–243.
7. Kazerooni EA, Armstrong MR, Amorosa JK, Hernandez D, Liebscher LA, Nath H, et al. ACR CT accreditation program and the lung cancer screening program designation. *J Am Coll Radiol.* 2016;13(2 Suppl):R30–34.
8. AAPM. Lung Cancer Screening CT Protocols Version 5.1.2019. Accessed April 22, 2021. https://www.aapm.org/pubs/CTProtocols/documents/LungCancerScreeningCT.pdf.
9. American College of Radiology. ACR Lung CT Screening Reporting & Data System (Lung-RADS). 2020. Accessed April 22, 2022. https://www.acr.org/Clinical-Resources/Reporting-and-Data-Systems/Lung-Rads.
10. Aramato SG, McLennan G, Bidaut L, et al. Data From LIDC-IDRI Chest CT Image Data Repository. The Cancer Imaging Archive. 2015. Accessed April 22, 2022.https://wiki.cancerimagingarchive.net/display/Public/LIDC-IDRI.
11. Armato III SG, McLennan G, Bidaut L, McNitt-Gray MF, Meyer CR, Reeves AP, et al. The Lung Image Database Consortium (LIDC) and Image Database Resource Initiative (IDRI): a completed reference database of lung nodules on CT scans. *Med Phys.* 2011;38(2):915–931.
12. Clark K, Vendt B, Smith K, Freymann J, Kirby J, Koppel P, et al. The Cancer Imaging Archive (TCIA): maintaining and operating a public information repository. *J Digit Imaging.* 2013;26(6):1045–1057.
13. Radiologic Society of North America. Quantitative Imaging Biomarker Alliance. 2020. Accessed October 30,2020. https://qibawiki.rsna.org/index.php/Profiles.
14. Milanese G, Eberhard M, Martini K, Vittoria De Martini I, Frauenfelder T. Vessel suppressed chest computed tomography for semi-automated volumetric measurements of solid pulmonary nodules. *Eur J Radiol.* 2018;101:97–102.
15. American College of Radiology. Lung-RADS Version 1.1.2019. Accessed 2020. https://www.acr.org/-/media/ACR/Files/RADS/Lung-RADS/LungRADSAssessmentCategoriesv1-1.pdf?la=en.
16. Zach JA, Newell Jr. JD, Schroeder J, Murphy JR, Curran-Everett D, Hoffman EA, et al. Quantitative computed tomography of the lungs and airways in healthy nonsmoking adults. *Invest Radiol.* 2012;47(10):596–602.
17. Wilson R, Devaraj A. Radiomics of pulmonary nodules and lung cancer. *Transl Lung Cancer Res.* 2017;6(1):86–91.
18. Ma J, Wang Q, Ren Y, et al. Automatic lung nodule classification with radiomics approach. *Proceedings of the SPIE.* 2016;9879:1117.
19. Lee SH, Lee SM, Goo JM, Kim KG, Kim YJ, Park CM. Usefulness of texture analysis in differentiating transient from persistent part-solid nodules(PSNs): a retrospective study. *PLoS One.* 2014;9(1):e85167.

CHAPTER 5

Using Reactive Machine AI to Derive Quantitative Lung CT Metrics of COPD, ILD, and COVID-19 Pneumonia

Introduction

This chapter will first review the basic structure of the human lung and use this information to explore the different QCT lung metrics that can be obtained from a single chest CT scan obtained at total lung capacity (TLC). A chest CT scan obtained at TLC and analyzed using lung CT AI can detect and assess lung density changes that occur in patients with emphysema from COPD, pulmonary inflammation and fibrosis in ILD, and acute viral pneumonia from COVID-19. The changes in lung density that result from these different diseases reflect important structural changes in the lung tissue that correlate with other measures of lung disease, such as clinical symptoms, exercise limitations, and pulmonary function testing. The successful application of lung CT AI to the assessment of diffuse lung diseases depends on the following four important steps: (1) quantitative chest CT protocol to acquire high-quality 3D CT images of both lungs, (2) segment the lungs from the rest of the thoracic anatomy, (3) extract quantitative CT metrics from the lung CT images and, (4) use the extracted QCT metrics to detect and assess normal and diseased lung tissue (Fig. 5.1).

Normal Lung Structure

The human lung is the largest visceral organ in the human body with a volume between 4 and 6 liters in normal adults. The lung is comprised mainly of air and water. The lung has high intrinsic contrast for x-ray CT imaging because the lung is 80% air and 20% water with HU values of −1000 HU and 0 HU, respectively. The high intrinsic contrast in the lung between water density and air density enables high-quality CT images of normal lung tissue, airways, and blood vessels.

There are 23 generations of airways from the trachea to the alveoli. The trachea is the first airway generation. There are two functional compartments of the lung airways: conducting airways, airway generations 1 to 16, airway generations 17 to 23, and gas diffusion (Fig. 5.2). The conducting airways transport air from the largest conducting airway, the trachea, to the smallest conducting airway the terminal bronchiole, generation 16. The terminal bronchial conducts air to the lung acinus, which is the largest gas exchanging unit of the lung. The structure of the acinus includes several generations of respiratory bronchioles, alveolar ducts, and alveoli (Fig. 5.3). The lung is designed to

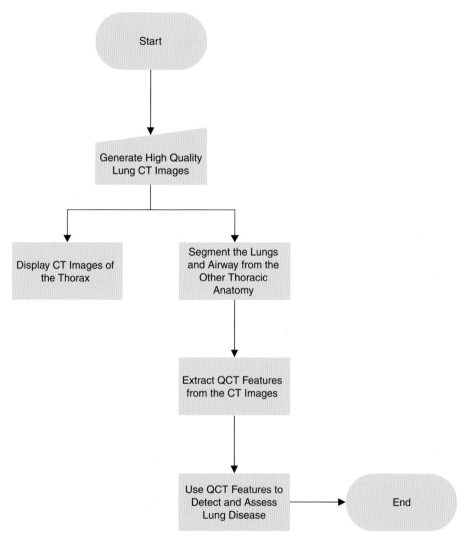

Fig. 5.1 Flow diagram outlining the important steps in a Reactive AI algorithm to assess a TLC lung CT scan for evidence of normal and diseased lung tissue.

provide a very efficient transfer of oxygen and carbon dioxide gases. The oxygen molecules in inspired air are transferred from the alveolar spaces to the red blood cells, and carbon dioxide is transferred from red blood cells to the alveolar air spaces. The essential structural features of the lung include the high surface to volume ratio of the lung structure, as well as the thin alveolar walls that enable a very efficient exchange of oxygen from the alveolar lumen into the capillary lumen within the wall of the alveolus, and the efficient exchange of carbon dioxide from the red blood cells in the capillary lumen into the alveolar space. The surface area of the alveolar walls in a human lung is the size of a tennis court, 140 m², but are folded into a very compact space 6 liters in size.[1] The normal thickness of the alveolar wall is about 2 microns.[1]

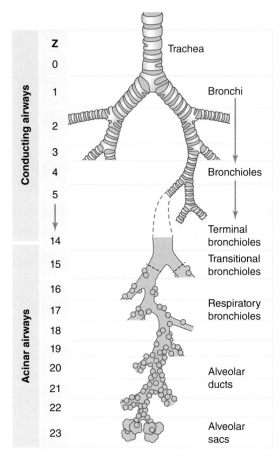

Fig. 5.2   Different generations of conducting and diffusion airways of the human lung.

QCT Scanning Protocol and Lung Segmentation

The first step in lung CT AI of diffuse lung disease is to obtain a quality 3D chest CT scan using an appropriate QCT scanning protocol that we described in detail in Chapter 3. In this chapter, we will discuss using a single TLC CT scan to assess normal and diseased lung structure. In Chapter 6, we will discuss how to obtain functional lung information by using both a TLC chest CT scan and an FRC/RV chest CT scan.

The second step is to automatically and consistently segment the lungs from the rest of the chest anatomy using a validated software program for this purpose. The computer algorithms that do this are quite sophisticated and use reactive AI, limited memory AI, or a combination of these AI levels.[2] These AI algorithms are designed to run automatically and are very efficient. Fig. 5.4 shows an axial, sagittal, and coronal chest CT image from a normal patient. Lower density is represented by darker gray colors and higher dense tissues with lighter gray colors. The low density of normal lung tissue reflects the fact that the normal lung is 80% air and 20% soft tissue (10% blood and 10% tissue).[1] The solid cylindrical branching soft tissue density structures in the lung are the arteries and veins.

Subdivisions of intrapulmonary airways

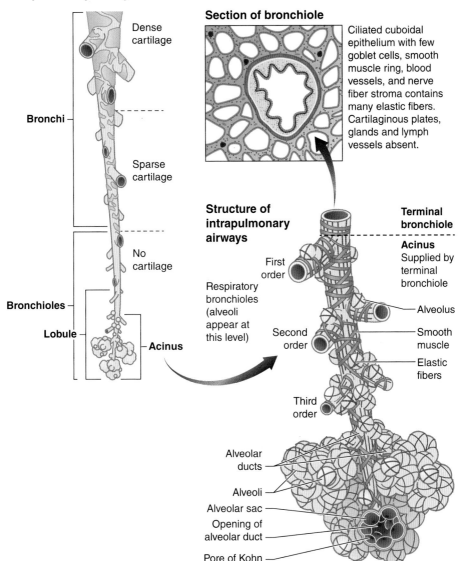

Section of bronchiole

Ciliated cuboidal epithelium with few goblet cells, smooth muscle ring, blood vessels, and nerve fiber stroma contains many elastic fibers. Cartilaginous plates, glands and lymph vessels absent.

Dense cartilage

Bronchi

Sparse cartilage

Structure of intrapulmonary airways

No cartilage

Respiratory bronchioles (alveoli appear at this level)

First order

Second order

Third order

Terminal bronchiole

Acinus Supplied by terminal bronchiole

Alveolus

Smooth muscle

Elastic fibers

Bronchioles

Lobule

Acinus

Alveolar ducts

Alveoli

Alveolar sac

Opening of alveolar duct

Pore of Kohn

Fig. 5.3 Terminal bronchiole, respiratory bronchioles, alveolar ducts, and alveoli that make up the pulmonary acinus of the lung as described in the text. The pulmonary acinus is the largest gas exchanging unit of the human lung.

The hollow cylindrical branching air-containing structures are the airways. Fig. 5.5 shows a 3D lung CT image after the image segmentation software has processed the original chest CT images.

The third step of lung CT AI to assess diffuse lung disease is to extract quantitative CT features from the segmented lung CT images. This can be used in step four to detect

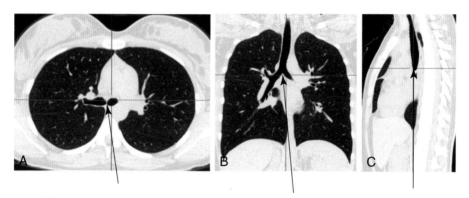

Fig. 5.4   (A) axial, (B) coronal, and (C) sagittal 2D planar images of the thorax at the level of the carina at the bifurcation of the trachea *(arrows)*. These images were displayed using a WW of 1500 HU and a WL of −500 HU. These WW and WL settings optimize the chest CT images for displaying the lung tissue for visual assessment.

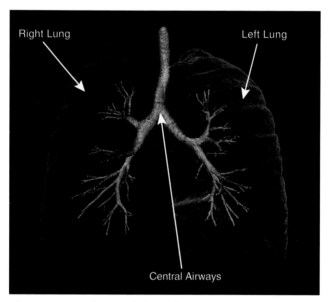

Fig. 5.5   3D semitransparent surface rendering of the lungs with only the trachea and lung tissue remaining. The rest of the chest anatomy (e.g., chest wall, spine, heart, aorta) has been removed. The large central pulmonary artery and veins have also been removed. The lung voxel histograms that we discuss in this chapter are derived from the lung portrayed here with the central airways and central pulmonary vessels removed. The airways and central pulmonary vessels are usually assessed separately. The central airways are discussed toward the end of Chapter 6 and the central pulmonary vessels are discussed in Chapter 8. (Courtesy of VIDA.)

and assess normal and diseased lung tissue. In this chapter, we will discuss straightforward reactive lung CT AI methods to derive CT features from the lung voxel histogram (Fig. 5.6). The fourth step of lung CT AI is to use the CT features derived in step three

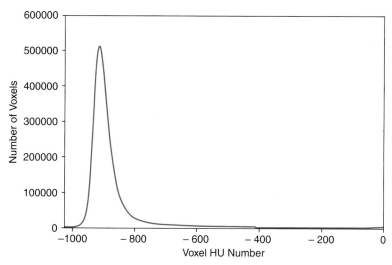

Fig. 5.6   TLC lung CT voxel histogram plot from a normal patient. The mean lung density is −860 HU in this normal patient.

to assess the presence and extent of diffuse lung disease. Normal lung density, decreased lung density from emphysema, and increased lung density from pulmonary fibrosis and pneumonia can be assessed using Reactive Lung CT AI.

Chronic Obstructive Pulmonary Disease (COPD) Induced Changes in Lung Structure

COPD first produces narrowing and destruction of small conducting airways before emphysema develops in the human lung.[3] The narrowing and destruction of small conducting airways increase the resistance to airflow in COPD. The progression of COPD can then produce emphysema in the lung. "Emphysema is defined as a condition of the lung characterized by abnormal, permanent enlargement of airspaces distal to the terminal bronchiole, accompanied by the destruction of alveolar walls, and without obvious lung fibrosis".[4] This enlargement of alveoli and the destruction of alveolar walls effectively reduces the available surface area for gas exchange per unit volume of lung tissue; therefore the efficiency of gas exchange in the lung is decreased in emphysema. The destruction of tissue in emphysema will decrease the density of lung tissue, and this can be detected and assessed using lung CT AI.

QUANTITATIVE CT METRICS OF LUNG DENSITY IN COPD

3D CT images of the lungs can be analyzed by looking at the location and individual values of the lung CT voxels in the lung. The simplest approach is to assess the lung CT voxel histogram of both lungs. The spatial information is lost in this approach if the voxel histograms of both lungs are combined. Fig. 5.6 shows the voxel histogram plot of normal lungs. Fig. 5.7 shows the voxel histogram plot of emphysematous lungs.

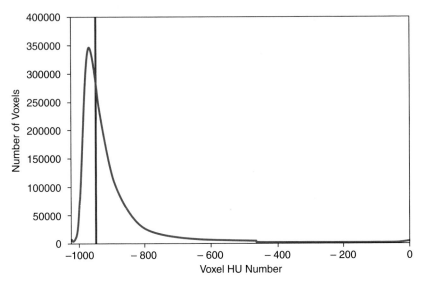

Fig. 5.7   TLC lung CT voxel histogram from a patient with severe emphysema. The mean lung density is −890 HU and the LAA$_{-950}$ is 39%. A vertical red line marks the −950 HU value.

Assessing features of the lung CT voxel histogram was one of the earliest methods of quantitatively assessing normal and diseased lung tissue.[5] The disadvantage of combining the CT lung voxels from both lungs is that the spatial information is lost. This can be overcome by assessing the CT voxel histogram at smaller scales. This has been done for individual lungs, lung lobes, sublobar segments, and individual voxels. The voxel-level completely preserves the spatial and CT voxel value information for each voxel, and can then be further processed with more powerful lung CT AI methods; more on this in Chapter 6. The following discussion will elaborate on different quantitative lung metrics that can be derived from the lung CT voxel histogram from a single TLC lung CT scan, and how they can be used to detect and assess normal and diseased lung tissue.

Mean Lung Density (MLD) for the Detection and Assessment of Emphysema

There are several ways to analyze the lung CT voxel histogram curve (Figs. 5.6 and 5.7) that can provide meaningful quantitative CT metrics of normal lung tissue and lung tissue with emphysema. Emphysema decreases the density of the lung tissue due to the destruction of alveolar walls and capillaries within those walls and also increases the volume of the lungs due to decreased elastic recoil of the lung tissue (Fig. 5.8). The decrease in lung tissue density in the emphysematous lung tissue, compared to normal lung tissue, can be detected by assessing the values of the lung CT voxels. The mean lung density (MLD) can be assessed by calculating the mean value of the lung CT voxels, and the CT determined MLD will decrease if there is emphysema in the lung. MLD density in normal subjects is greater than the MLD in patients with emphysema; an early research study reported this in 1982.[5] The histogram curves from a normal lung and a lung with a lot of emphysema are shown in Figs. 5.6 and 5.7. The MLD is indicated in

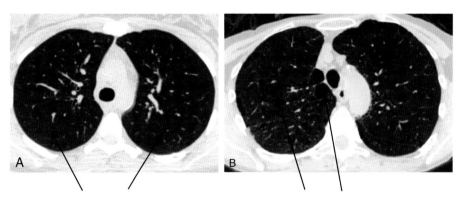

Fig. 5.8 Two axial chest CT images. **(A)** Normal lung with normal lung density *(arrows)*. **(B)** Focal areas of decreased density *(arrows)* that are due to tissue destruction from emphysema.

these figures and you can see that the emphysematous lung has a mean lung density that is lower than the mean MLD of a normal lung. You can also appreciate that the shape of the histogram has also changed. Mean lung density, standard deviation, skewness, and kurtosis of the lung CT voxel histogram curve will change between normal lung and emphysematous lung, and also between normal lung and pulmonary fibrosis from ILD. This will be discussed further in this chapter.

Low Attenuating Area (LAA) for the Detection and Assessment of Emphysema

Another approach to assessing the lung CT voxel histogram for the presence or absence of emphysema is to use a threshold approach where the number of voxels below a certain voxel value in HU is assessed. There are two popular approaches to assessing the number of lung CT voxels below a certain threshold. The first approach picks a fixed voxel value and assesses the number of lung CT voxels that fall below this voxel value or threshold. This is referred to as the density mask, or low attenuating area (LAA) method, and is usually expressed as a percentage of lung CT voxels that are less than the threshold. The currently accepted LAA threshold for severe emphysema is −950 HU and expressed as LAA_{-950} (Fig. 5.7). The second approach picks a fixed fraction or percentage of low attenuating voxels (e.g., 15%) in the lung CT voxel histogram and then assesses the lung CT voxel value that separates the lowest 15% of lung voxel values from the remaining higher 85% of voxel values. The currently accepted percentile method is the 15th percentile method.

In 1988 Muller et al. reported their results using an LAA thresholding method they described as the "Density Mask" technique to detect and assess emphysema.[6] The density mask software in this study measures the number of lung voxels less than a certain threshold. The study looked at threshold values of −900 HU, −910 HU, and −920 HU; the −910 HU threshold gave the best results in this study. There were 28 subjects in this study. The CT scans were obtained on a single row fan-beam detector array, third-generation axial CT scanner, GE 9800. The entire lung was scanned using 10-mm-thick axial images obtained 10 mm apart, contiguous images of the whole lungs. Each of the subjects was referred for resection of their lung cancers after their CT scans. The study assessed visual evidence of emphysema, quantitative CT evidence of emphysema looking at the amount of lung, >-910 HU, and pathologic evidence of emphysema on the resected lung specimens. The same area of lung was examined by visual CT, quantitative CT, and pathological assessment of the lung. There was excellent agreement between all three methods. Intravenous contrast material was administered to each subject and this may have raised the optimal cutoff point in this study.

One of the quantitative CT challenges for assessing emphysema in the 1990s was trying to determine the optimal threshold for the LAA method. There were two key papers published in 1995 and 1996 by Gevenois et al. that established the optimal LAA threshold voxel value was -950 HU.[7,8] The LAA$_{-950}$ that was established by Gevenois is still used today.[9] The optimal LAA threshold is also a function of the voxel size and the reconstruction kernel. The studies by Gevenois used a voxel that was approximately $1\,mm \times 1\,mm \times 1\,mm$, whereas the study by Mueller, used a voxel size of approximately $10\,mm \times 10\,mm \times 10\,mm$.[6] The smaller the voxel size the better small emphysematous lesions, $<5\,mm$, can be detected and a lower LAA threshold value is justified.

Let us look more closely at the two studies by Gevenois that concluded the optimal LAA threshold for emphysema was -950 HU.[7,8] These two important studies looked at the correlation between macroscopic and microscopic pathologic evidence of emphysema and the QCT LAA -950 metric.[7,8] The first study, in 1995, showed an excellent correlation between the area of emphysema on macroscopic horizontally/axially sectioned lung pathology specimens and the QCT LAA -950 HU metric for emphysema on high-resolution CT images of the lungs, xyz-plane resolution $<2\,mm$. The axial pathology specimens were macroscopic tissue sections obtained every 1 to 2 cm from the resected lobe(s) or lung. In this study, 1.25 mm axial CT images of the lungs were obtained at 1-cm intervals, and these were assessed for emphysema using the LAA method where the fraction of lung voxels, >-950 HU, is expressed as a percent (e.g., LAA$_{-950}$ = 15%). This study looked at a number of thresholds from -900 HU to -970 HU. The LAA -950 HU level had the best agreement with the macroscopic scores for emphysema on the axial pathology specimens of the lungs.

The second paper, published in 1996, examined the lung tissue obtained in the 1995 paper using microscopic methods of assessing normal lung tissue and emphysematous lung tissue.[8] This included assessing the mean perimeter (MP) of the alveoli and alveolar ducts of 35 randomly selected microscopic fields, 25× magnification, and the mean interwall distance (MIWD) of alveoli and alveolar ducts within the 35 randomly selected fields. The randomly selected microscopic sections were assessed by experienced pathologists to classify them into normal lung or emphysematous lung. The MP and MIWD values were correlated with the CT LAA values for a range of LAA thresholds from -900 HU to -970 HU by 10 HU increments. The strongest correlation between MP and MIWD was the LAA set at -950 HU. There were multiple strong correlations between the MP and MIWD values and measures of the patient's pulmonary function tests, with the strongest correlations being between DLCO/VA percent predicted and MP, MIWD, and Macroscopic evidence of emphysema. Setting the LAA threshold to -950 HU is now generally accepted as the best threshold value to use in an LAA method for the detection and assessment of emphysema on a TLC chest CT scan.

15th Percentile Method for the Detection and Assessment of Emphysema

The 15th percentile method of assessing the lung CT voxel histogram for evidence of emphysema picks a fixed fraction or percentage of low attenuating voxels (e.g., 15%) of the lung CT voxel histogram, and then assesses the lung CT voxel value that separates the lowest 15% of lung voxel values from the remaining higher 85% of voxel values. The percentile method was first introduced by Gould et al. in 1988.[10]

Gould et al. described in 1988 the close correlation of low-density areas seen on chest CT with both macroscopic and microscopic measures of emphysema.[10] The microscopic assessment of emphysema included measuring the surface area of distal airspace walls (e.g., alveolar walls) to the unit lung volume ratio (AWUV) of the lung in patients with mild to moderate emphysema who had preoperative CT scans and pulmonary function testing and then subsequently underwent lobe or lung resection for nonsmall cell lung cancer, which is a frequent unfortunate complication in heavy smokers with and without COPD. There was a strong correlation in this study between the EMI CT number of the fifth percentile and microscopic evidence of emphysema using the mean AWUV. There was also a strong correlation between the mean AWUV and pulmonary function tests. These results established that assessing the lung CT voxel histogram using the percentile method is a valid noninvasive test to detect and assess emphysema in COPD patients.[10] There are several points worth discussing further in regards to this early high impact paper. First, the CT scanner used was an EMI 5005 CT scanner that obtained a 1.5 mm × 1.5 mm × 13 mm, axial image of the thorax with a scanning time of 17 seconds. The authors indicated that each CT image was obtained within 500 mL of TLC, though it is not clear how this was determined. The EMI unit is half the value of the Hounsfield unit previously discussed in this section. In this study by Gould, they recommended viewing the lung tissue for emphysema by highlighting the voxels in the CT image between −500 EMI units and −450 EMI units. This can be expressed as LAA using EMI units rather than HU units (e.g., $LAA_{-450EMI}$). This would correspond to −1000 HU and −900 HU. This can be viewed as a LAA_{-900HU} approach to assessing emphysema, as discussed in the LAA section on detection and assessment of emphysema. Gould did not assess the $LAA_{-450EMI}$ quantitatively. The fifth percentile method in this study would translate to the 10% method using HU units for the voxel histogram rather than the EMI units of the original paper. Gould's 1988 paper found that the CT voxel fifth percentile method for the assessment of emphysema was highly correlated to the mean AWUV, R = −0.63. Gould also showed that the mean AWUV was highly correlated with the DLCO/Va, R = 0.66. The authors did not assess the correlation of the $LAA_{-450EMI}$ with mean AWUV. We do not know why LAA was not investigated. The fifth percentile number varied from −479 EMI to −414 EMI units or −958 HU to −828 HU. The authors conclude that the results of their study indicate that CT measures of lung density and DLCO/VA in the living patient can objectively assess the alveolar surface to volume ratio, and can also localize spatially those portions of the lung that are contributing to the loss of tissue and expansion of airspaces which the DLCO/VA cannot. This paper was written in 1988 and this book is being written in 2020; we are now at the point of using CT measures of lung density as an objective way to assess the decreasing alveolar surface to volume ratio that occurs in COPD subjects with emphysema in routine clinical care of patients. The path was clear several decades ago, but many technological advances in lung CT AI were necessary before the automatic assessment of the lung CT voxel histogram could be integrated into routine clinical care, see Chapter 9.

The 15th percentile method was used by Dirksen et al. in the late 1990s to build on the work of Gould, that we have just described.[11,12] Dirksen's work used improvements in CT scanner technology to obtain CT scans of the entire lung in a single breath-hold. This was made possible by using the spiral CT scanning mode that was not available to Gould in the late 1980s.

The 15th percentile method determines the CT number in HU that determines the point in the lung voxel histogram curve where 15% of the lung voxels are less than this number and 85% are greater than this number. The idea here is that as emphysematous lung tissue replaces normal lung tissue, the value of the Perc15 HU value will shift toward lower values. There was a detailed study looking at LAA cutoffs and percent cutoffs by Dirksen; they showed the optimal percentile for the percentile method was the 12th percentile and that the 12th percentile method performed better than LAA using level -930 HU in assessing longitudinal changes in the amount of emphysema present in subjects with alpha-1 antitrypsin deficiency (A1AD).[12] This study looked at the percentiles from 1% to 50% by 1% increments and found the best results were in the range of 10% to 20%. A subsequent study (see Chapter 3) by Dirksen looking at patients with A1AD for a period of 3 years used the 15th percentile method to detect and assess A1AD related emphysematous lung tissue.[11] Dirksen reported in 1999 that quantitative CT using the 15th percentile point of the lung density histogram showed decreased progression of A1AD induced emphysema in A1AD patients who were receiving monthly intravenous augmentation therapy with human alpha-AT.[11] The quantitative CT results were much more sensitive than monitoring decreases in airflow measured using the forced expiratory volume in one second, FEV1. This was a turning point in the development of lung CT AI using quantitative CT metrics, such as the 15th percentile method, because now quantitative lung CT was doing something noninvasively that visual lung CT and pulmonary physiological measures of lung function could not do.

Clinical Value of Using Lung CT AI in Patients with Environmental Exposure to Cigarette Smoke

Both LAA_{-950} and the 15th percentile methods are two quantitative CT metrics that were both developed some time ago and persist today as the two favored methods of assessing the emphysema-related structural changes in the lung that reduce lung density. The LAA_{-950} and the 15th percentile are derived from the lung voxel histogram curves from a single chest CT scan obtained at TLC.[9,13] There has been considerable research done looking at patients with COPD and determining what the clinical benefit of lung CT AI is in COPD patients.

CLINICAL BENEFIT OF LAA_{-950}

The COPD Genetic Epidemiology study (COPDGene) is a large, 10,263 subjects enrolled in phase 1, ongoing multicenter NIH-funded research study that began in 2007. Recently the study has reported results using the LAA_{-950} method of the lung CT voxel histogram to detect and assess emphysema at baseline and 5 years.[9,14]

> **BOX 5.1 ■ The Four Novel COPDGene COPD Criteria**
>
> 1. Exposure
>   - 10-pack-year or more smoking history
> 2. Symptoms
>   - mMRC dyspnea score of ≥ 2 or chronic bronchitis
> 3. CT Structural Abnormality
>   - LAA_{-950} $\geq 5\%$ on a TLC chest CT scan (QCT structural measure of emphysema); or
>   - LAA_{-856} $\geq 15\%$ on expiratory CT scan (QCT functional measure of air trapping); or
>   - Pi10 ≥ 2.5 mm (QCT evidence of airway wall remodeling
> 4. Spirometry Evidence of COPD
>   - FEV1/FVC >0.70; or
>   - FEV1% predicted $>80\%$

In the phase 1 study, 8784 subjects were evaluated to assess subsequent mortality risk. Five years later, 4925 returning subjects who were studied at baseline in the phase 1 study were evaluated to assess the risk of decline in FEV1. The current method of diagnosing COPD requires postbronchodilator pulmonary function testing in a patient suspected of having COPD by using Spirometry to assess airflow, FEV1, lung volume, FVC, and the ratio of FEV1/FVC to make the diagnosis of COPD.[9,15] The diagnosis of COPD requires that the FEV1/FVC ratio is less than 0.70.[15]

A substantial number of patients with COPD manifest respiratory symptoms and CT structural evidence of COPD, suggesting COPD, before they develop an FEV1/FVC ratio less than 0.70.[9] The COPDGene study has recently shown that these same patients are at increased risk of death and progressive decline in their FEV1/FVC ratio, and FEV1 percent predicted.[9] The COPDGene study used the following four novel criteria to diagnose COPD and to assess the impact of these criteria on COPD progression and mortality: "Exposure, Symptoms, CT Structural Abnormality, Spirometry" (Box 5.1).[9] Exposure was defined as having a 10-pack-year or greater smoking history.[9] Symptoms were defined as self-reporting a modified Medical Council (mMRC) dyspnea score of 2 or greater, and/ or chronic bronchitis (self-reported chronic cough and phlegm).[9] CT structural abnormality was defined as having one or more of the following: LAA_{-950} equal to 5% or greater on a TLC chest CT scan (QCT structural measure of Emphysema), LAA_{-856} equal to or greater than 15% on expiratory CT scan (QCT functional measure of air trapping), Pi10 equal to 2.5 mm or greater (QCT structural measure of airway wall thickening).[9] Spirometry evidence of COPD was defined as having an FEV1/FVC less than 0.70 and/or an FEV1 percentage predicted less than 80%.[9] This COPDGene study proposed a scheme of assessing subjects with respiratory symptoms suspicious of COPD by placing them into one of eight categories, A thru H, using the four novel criteria just described: Exposure, Symptoms, CT Structural Abnormalities, Spirometry (Box 5.2).[9] Category A is a patient with significant exposure to cigarette smoke. Category B is a patient with significant exposure to cigarette smoke and QCT evidence of COPD. Category C is a patient with significant exposure to cigarette smoke and clinical symptoms of COPD. Category D is a patient with significant exposure to cigarette smoke and abnormal spirometry with FEV1/FVC ratio less than 0.70 and/or FEV1 percent predicted less than 80%. Category E is a patient

---

BOX 5.2 ■ Eight COPDGene Patient Categories for COPD

A. Exposure
B. Exposure + CT Structural Abnormality
C. Exposure + Symptoms
D. Exposure + Spirometry Evidence of COPD
E. Exposure + Symptoms + CT Structural Abnormality
F. Exposure + Symptoms + Spirometry Evidence of COPD
G. Exposure + CT Structural Abnormality + Spirometry Evidence of COPD
H. Exposure + Symptoms + CT Structural Abnormality + Spirometry Evidence of COPD

BOX 5.3 ■ Four COPDGene Classes of COPD

1. No COPD
　■ Category A patients
2. Possible COPD
　■ Category B, C, D patients
3. Probable COPD
　■ Category E, F, G patients
4. Definite COPD
　■ Category H patients

---

with significant exposure to cigarette smoke, QCT evidence of COPD, and clinical symptoms of COPD. Category F, is a patient with significant exposure to cigarette smoke, clinical symptoms of COPD, and abnormal spirometry with FEV1/FVC ratio less than 0.70 and/or FEV1 percent predicted less than 80%. Category G, is a patient with significant exposure to cigarette smoke, QCT evidence of COPD, and abnormal spirometry with FEV1/FVC ratio less than 0.70 and/or FEV1 percent predicted less than 80%. Category H is a patient with significant exposure to cigarette smoke, QCT evidence of COPD, clinical symptoms of COPD, and abnormal spirometry with FEV1/FVC ratio less than 0.70 and/or FEV1 percent predicted less than 80%. Categories A thru H are summarized in Box 5.2.

This COPDGene study then grouped the eight categories above into four COPDGene 2019 Classes of COPD: No COPD, Possible COPD, Probable COPD, and Definite COPD. Grouping the eight categories into these four classes of COPD was done by assessing the odds of a change in FEV1 greater than 350 mL over a 5 year period and the hazard ratio for all-cause mortality over 5 years. Category A subjects were classified as No COPD. Category B, C, and D subjects were classified as Possible COPD. Category E, F, and G subjects were classified as Probable COPD. Category H subjects were classified as Definite COPD (Box 5.3).[9]

This is a very important study validating the value of lung CT AI in the assessment of patients suspected of having COPD. The COPDGene 2019 approach to diagnosing COPD would increase the number of patients diagnosed earlier in the course of their COPD illness by including QCT in the diagnosis of COPD.[9] Definite COPD needs QCT evidence of COPD. Possible COPD can be detected and assessed using QCT evidence of COPD when there are no clinical symptoms and normal spirometry. Probable

COPD can be detected and assessed using QCT evidence of COPD when there is either normal spirometry or no clinical symptoms. There is a high value in using lung CT AI in the routine clinical assessment of patients with and without respiratory symptoms, but with known or unknown exposure to significant amounts of cigarette smoke. Before QCT can be required in the diagnosis of COPD, lung CT AI methods must be available and efficient in the clinical practice of lung CT imaging. It is not surprising that the results of this study and other similar studies have motivated lung CT AI companies to introduce software tools into the clinical practice of lung CT imaging to improve the detection and assessment of patients with COPD. This will be discussed more in Chapter 9.

Interstitial Lung Disease (ILD) Induced Changes in Lung Structure

There are four anatomic divisions of the lung that can be altered in acute and chronic diseases of the lung, such as acute pneumonia and chronic interstitial pneumonia, which can increase the density of the lungs. These four anatomic divisions include the alveolar space, interstitial space, airways, and pulmonary vessels. The components of this increased soft tissue density include water, proliferation of type 2 pneumocytes, immune cells, and extracellular matrix. The density of the lung increases due to increases in tissue volume and decreases in air volume.

In acute pneumonia produced by COVID-19, other viral pneumonia, bacterial pneumonia, fungal and parasitic pneumonia, the initial increase in lung density occurs primarily in the alveolar lumen and alveolar wall. There is an increase in water, plasma proteins, and immune cells in these areas. These increases in soft tissue elements in the alveolar lumen, which normally contains air, produce a marked increase in lung density in the alveolar lumen, and this process appears as ground-glass opacities if it is incomplete and as consolidation, if it is complete. When the lung tissue has consolidation there is no air left in the alveolar lumen so the pulmonary vessels and airway walls are not visible, but the lumen of the airways may persist. The presence of airway lumens surrounded by abnormally high lung density tissue density is called air bronchograms and help to identify consolidation. Incomplete alveolar lumen filling where there are still identifiable pulmonary vessels and airway walls is called ground-glass opacity. Pure ground-glass opacity does not have any additional texture features, such as reticulations from intralobular and interlobular septal thickening, dilated airways, and honeycomb cysts. Fig. 5.9 shows an example of increased lung density, ground–glass, and reticular opacities due to COVID-19 viral pneumonia. Fig. 5.10 shows an example of focal consolidation from COVID-19 pneumonia.

Chronic interstitial pneumonia or chronic ILD is produced by previous acute pneumonia, connective tissue disease, hypersensitivity pneumonitis, and occupational lung disease, such as silicosis. There may be no known etiology, also termed idiopathic or cryptogenic. Idiopathic pulmonary fibrosis (IPF) is a common cause of chronic interstitial pneumonia where currently there is no known etiology (Fig. 5.11). Cryptogenic organizing pneumonia is another cause of chronic ILD where there is no known etiology. The increase in lung density in IPF occurs primarily by a decrease in the size of the alveolar lumen with increased fibrotic tissue in the alveolar walls and decreased intravascular volume, which is not easily reversible. Cryptogenic organizing pneumonia has increases of fibrotic tissue in the alveolar lumen and alveolar walls.

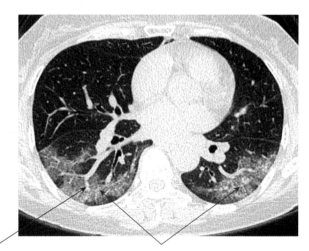

Fig. 5.9   Axial chest CT image of a patient with COVID-19 viral pneumonia. Note the increase in lung density due to bilateral, lower lobe, peripheral and dorsal ground–glass, and reticular opacities *(red arrows)*. There is moderate increase in lung density. Pulmonary vessels can still be identified in the areas of increased density *(blue arrow)*.

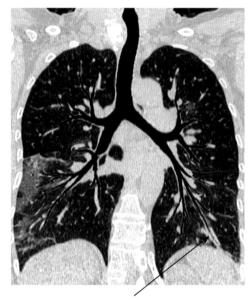

Fig. 5.10   tMPR lung CT image from a COVID-19 viral pneumonia patient demonstrates increased lung density from focal consolidation in the left lower lobe with an air bronchogram *(arrow)*. Ximus conscrita L.

LUNG DENSITY, VOLUMES, SPECIFIC AIR AND TISSUE VOLUMES IN IPF

The paper by Coxson et al. in 1997 evaluated normal control lungs with IPF lungs showed that CT scans and pathology examination of the lung tissue from surgical resections in the control subjects and surgical biopsies in the IPF patients, exhibited a marked

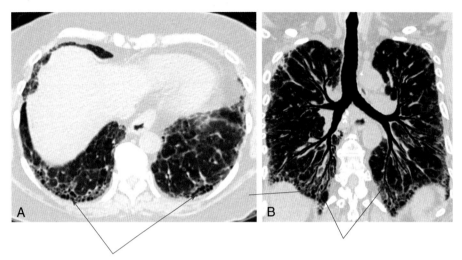

Fig. 5.11   (A) axial lung CT and (B) coronal tMPR lung CT in a patient with ILD from IPF. Traction bronchiectasis *(blue arrows,* ***B****)* and honeycombing *(red arrows,* ***A*** *and* ***B****)* are present.

decrease in air volume with preservation of tissue volume and tissue weight in the IPF patients compared to controls.[16]

The CT scans for the control subjects were obtained using a GE Highlight Advantage CT scanner at St Paul's Hospital, Vancouver, British Columbia. The scanning protocol used 120 kVp, 100 mA, 2-second scan time, 10-mm-slice thickness, and contiguous images of the entire right and left lungs prior to surgical resection or surgical lung biopsy. The CT data were transferred to a workstation in the Pulmonary Research Laboratory in Vancouver for x-ray attenuation value analysis. The IPF subjects were scanned on the C-100 Imatron electron beam CT scanner at the University of Iowa, Iowa City, Iowa. This scanning protocol used 130 kVp, 640 mA, 0.6-second scan time, 3-mm-slice thickness, and 20 mm gaps between slices. The CT images were printed on film and sent to the Pulmonary Research Laboratory in Vancouver, and the images from the film were transferred to a computer workstation for further analysis of the x-ray attenuation values. A custom computer program was developed to analyze the CT images of both the control subjects and the IPF subjects. This software program segmented the lungs from the rest of the thoracic anatomy and then calculated the lung volumes by summing up the volume of each voxel in the lungs. The mean CT attenuation in HU of each voxel was calculated and converted to gravimetric density, which is grams per millimeter, g/mL, by adding 1000 to the CT number in HU and then dividing this sum by 1000. Water is (0 HU + 1000)/1000 = 1.0 g/mL. The weight of the lung was determined by multiplying the volume of the lung by its mean density, both determined from the CT scan. The authors then convert the lung density measures to specific volumes which is the reciprocal of lung density, specific volume expressed as mL (gas)/g(tissue). Frequency histogram plots of the specific volumes of the control lung values and the IPF values were performed and compared. Tissue density is assumed to be 1.065 g/mL in this work.

The comparison between the CT lung analysis and the microscopic tissue analysis was done by obtaining the volume fraction of tissue and air determined from the CT scans and comparing this to the volume fraction of tissue and air determined by microscopic analysis. For example, the volume fraction of tissue from the CT scan was determined by this formula:

Vv (CT Tissue) = specific volume of tissue (assumed value 0.939 mL/g) /specific volume of total lung, mL/g, (determined by CT).

Similarly, the volume fraction of air from the CT scan was determined by this formula:

Vv (CT Air) = specific volume of air/

specific volume of total lung, mL/g, (determined by CT).

The surface-to-volume ratio decreased from a mean of 110 square meters in control subjects to 30 square meters in IPF subjects. The thickness of the alveolar walls increased from 8 microns to 97 microns. They point out that the process in IPF involves the collapse of the alveoli onto alveolar ducts which leads to a marked decrease in air volume, surface-to-volume ratio, and thickening of the alveolar walls. The increase in CT density is related to decreases in the air volume fraction of the lung and not due to significant increases in the tissue volume fraction.

This study was a great advancement in the validation of lung CT AI-derived lung volumes and CT-derived density and specific volume measurements in the assessment of patients with ILD from IPF with previously validated methods of microscopic tissue fixation and analysis.[16]

HISTOGRAM MEASURES OF ILD—MLD, SKEWNESS, KURTOSIS

Best et al. in 2003 published work showing that several CT metrics of ILD in IPF subjects could be derived from the CT voxel histogram curve (Fig. 5.12).

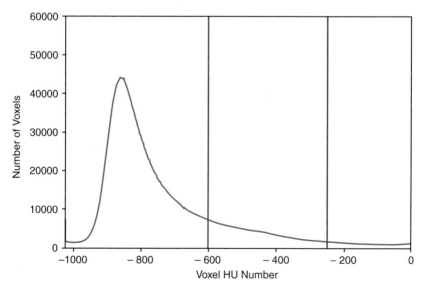

Fig. 5.12 Voxel histogram from a patient with ILD from IPF. The range of voxel values between −600 HU and −250 HU are marked with vertical red lines. The mean lung density (MLD) is −736 HU and the percent high attenuation area (%HAA) is 15%.

These measures included mean lung density, skewness, and kurtosis, and were shown to have moderate correlations to lung function measured by pulmonary function testing.[17] The lung function testing included measures of airflow, FEV1 and FVC, TLC, and DLCO. There were 144 subjects in this study. The subjects were a part of another study looking at the effectiveness of interferon-gamma in the treatment of IPF. The lungs were segmented using a semiautomated method that assumed an upper lung density threshold of −200 HU. An attenuation correction was applied to the CT image data. The most powerful predictor of pulmonary function among the QCT metrics was the kurtosis of the CT lung voxel histogram curve.

Similarly, in 2008, Best et al. showed that the quantitative CT metrics of mean lung density, skewness, and kurtosis showed progression of lung disease in 95 IPF subjects that were examined at baseline and after 12 months.[17] Pulmonary function testing, visual assessment of the CT images for ground-glass opacities, and pulmonary fibrosis were also performed in this study. Visual evidence of pulmonary fibrosis and FVC correlated with short-term mortality in a multivariable analysis.

PERCENT HIGH ATTENUATING AREAS (%HAA) IN ILD

Podolanczuk et al. in 2016 reported results using a quantitative CT lung metric referred to as the percent high attenuating areas (%HAA) to assess preclinical evidence of interstitial lung abnormalities in a middle-aged and older adult community-dwelling population.[18] The %HAA is defined as the amount of lung that is between −600 HU and −250 HU. The %HAA represents increases in lung densities, as opposed to the LAA, previously described in this chapter, reports on decreases in lung density. The amount of HAA in this study was shown to be associated with increased serum levels of interleukin six, IL-6, and matrix metalloproteinase seven, MMP-7, which are markers of lung tissue inflammation and lung tissue extracellular matrix remodeling respectively. HAA was also associated with decreases in forced vital capacity (FVC), decreased exercise capacity, increased odds of visual evidence of interstitial lung abnormalities (ILA) at 10-year follow-up, and an increase in mortality rate. The study concluded that the HAA QCT metric was a valid quantitative CT phenotype of subclinical lung injury and lung inflammation and that it may be a precursor to subclinical ILD. %HAA can be used to assess early, as well as, more advanced cases of ILD.

QCT of COVID-19 Acute Viral Pneumonia

The COVID-19 pandemic caused by the Severe Acute Respiratory Corona Virus 2, SAR Cov-2, affecting the entire world, is still ongoing at the time of this writing, December 2021. The typical COVID-19 viral pneumonia appearance on chest CT scans is that of bilateral, lower lobe, peripheral ground-glass, and consolidative opacities (Figs. 5.9 and 5.10).[19] Reactive machine lung CT AI methods have been used to detect and assess COVID-19 pneumonia on chest CT scans.[20]

Colombi et al. reported in 2020 that assessing the amount of well-aerated lung using visual lung CT or lung CT AI in patients with confirmed COVID-19 viral pneumonia, were better predictors of ICU admission or death when compared to nonimaging clinical parameters.[20] Each of the 236 patients in this study had a positive RT-PCR test for COVID-19, positive visual CT findings for viral pneumonia, and a complete set of relevant clinical parameters.[20] Both the visual and lung CT AI approaches assessed the amount of a normally aerated lung. These were both expressed as a percentage of the total lung.

The lung CT AI method first segments the normal lungs from the rest of the thoracic anatomy. Then the percent of the lung CT voxels between −950 HU and −700 HU are used to calculate the percentage of a normally aerated lung, %S-WAL. The absolute volume of a normally aerated lung is also calculated, VOL-WAL. The outcomes of the patient's hospitalization were used to group the patients into two categories: (1) alive and discharged without admission to the ICU, Alive/No ICU, (2) admitted to the ICU and/or died, ICU/Death.

The median value of the %S-WAL of the ICU/Death patient group was 57%. The median value of the %S-WAL of the Alive/No ICU patient group was 78%. The median value of the VOL-WAL in the ICU/Death patient group was 3.4 liters, and in the Alive/No ICU patient group was 2.3 liters. Multivariable logistic regression model analysis looking at independent predictors that the patient would be in the ICU/Death group showed that the best clinical predictors of ICU/Death were cardiovascular comorbidities and age >68 years. This same model showed that both %S-WAL and VOL-WAL were independent predictors of ICU/Death. If the amount of well-aerated lung, %S-WAL, was less than 71%, the odds that the patient would be in the ICU/Death group increased by 3.7. If the volume of well-aerated lung, VOL-WAL, was less than 2.9 liters, the odds that the patient would be in the ICU/Death group increased by 2.6.[20]

Summary

In this chapter, we have seen that using lung CT AI to assess lung disease using a single TLC chest CT scan is helpful in detecting and quantitating the amount of abnormal structural change in the lung from both emphysema, pulmonary fibrosis, and viral pneumonia. In the next chapter, we will explore the application of lung CT AI to assess lung ventilation using TLC and residual volume (RV) chest CT scans.

References

1. Knudsen L, Ochs M. The micromechanics of lung alveoli: structure and function of surfactant and tissue components. *Histochem Cell Biol.* 2018;150(6):661–676.
2. Mansoor A, Bagci U, Foster B, Xu Z, Papadakis GZ, Folio LR, et al. Segmentation and image analysis of abnormal lungs at CT: current approaches, challenges, and future trends. *Radiographics.* 2015;35(4):1056–1076.
3. McDonough JE, Yuan R, Suzuki M, Seyednejad N, Elliott WM, Sanchez PG, et al. Small-airway obstruction and emphysema in chronic obstructive pulmonary disease. *N Engl J Med.* 2011;365(17):1567–1575.
4. Snider GL, Kleinerman J, Thurlbeck WM, Bengali ZH. The definition of emphysema. Report of a National Heart, Lung, and Blood Institute, Division of Lung Diseases workshop. *Am Rev Respir Dis.* 1985;132(1):182–185.
5. Goddard PR, Nicholson EM, Laszlo G, Watt I. Computed tomography in pulmonary emphysema. *Clin Radiol.* 1982;33(4):379–387.
6. Muller NL, Staples CA, Miller RR, Abboud RT. "Density mask". An objective method to quantitate emphysema using computed tomography. *Chest.* 1988;94(4):782–787.

7. Gevenois PA, de Maertelaer V, De Vuyst P, Zanen J, Yernault JC. Comparison of computed density and macroscopic morphometry in pulmonary emphysema. *Am J Respir Crit Care Med.* 1995;152(2):653–657.

8. Gevenois PA, De Vuyst P, de Maertelaer V, Zanen J, Jacobovitz D, Cosio MG, et al. Comparison of computed density and microscopic morphometry in pulmonary emphysema. *Am J Respir Crit Care Med.* 1996;154(1):187–192.

9. Lowe KE, Regan EA, Anzueto A, Austin E, Austin JHM, Beaty TH, et al. COPDGene® 2019: Redefining the diagnosis of chronic obstructive pulmonary disease. *Chronic Obstr Pulm Dis.* 2019;6(5):384–399.

10. Gould GA, MacNee W, McLean A, Warren PM, Redpath A, Best JJ, et al. CT measurements of lung density in life can quantitate distal airspace enlargement—an essential defining feature of human emphysema. *Am Rev Respir Dis.* 1988;137(2):380–392.

11. Dirksen A, Dijkman JH, Madsen F, Stoel B, Hutchison DC, Ulrik CS, et al. A randomized clinical trial of alpha(1)-antitrypsin augmentation therapy. *Am J Respir Crit Care Med.* 1999;160(5 Pt 1):1468–1472.

12. Dirksen A, Friis M, Olesen KP, Skovgaard LT, Sorensen K. Progress of emphysema in severe alpha 1-antitrypsin deficiency as assessed by annual CT. *Acta Radiol.* 1997;38(5):826–832.

13. Pompe E, Strand M, van Rikxoort EM, Hoffman EA, Barr RG, Charbonnier JP, et al. Five-year progression of emphysema and air trapping at CT in smokers with and those without chronic obstructive pulmonary disease: Results from the COPDGene Study. *Radiology.* 2020 https://doi.org/10.1148/radiol.2020191429.

14. Regan EA, Hokanson JE, Murphy JR, Make B, Lynch DA, Beaty TH, et al. Genetic epidemiology of COPD (COPDGene) study design. *COPD.* 2010;7(1):32–43.

15. Vogelmeier CF, Criner GJ, Martinez FJ, Anzueto A, Barnes PJ, Bourbeau J, et al. Global strategy for the diagnosis, management, and prevention of chronic obstructive lung disease 2017 Report. GOLD Executive Summary. *Am J Respir Crit Care Med.* 2017;195(5):557–582.

16. Coxson HO, Hogg JC, Mayo JR, Behzad H, Whittall KP, Schwartz DA, et al. Quantification of idiopathic pulmonary fibrosis using computed tomography and histology. *Am J Respir Crit Care Med.* 1997;155(5):1649–1656.

17. Best AC, Lynch AM, Bozic CM, Miller D, Grunwald GK, Lynch DA. Quantitative CT indexes in idiopathic pulmonary fibrosis: relationship with physiologic impairment. *Radiology.* 2003;228(2):407–414.

18. Podolanczuk AJ, Oelsner EC, Barr RG, Hoffman EA, Armstrong HF, Austin JH, et al. High attenuation areas on chest computed tomography in community-dwelling adults: the MESA study. *Eur Respir J.* 2016;48(5):1442–1452.

19. Bernheim A, Mei X, Huang M, Yang Y, Fayad ZA, Zhang N, et al. Chest CT findings in coronavirus disease-19 (COVID-19): Relationship to duration of infection. *Radiology.* 2020 https://doi.org/10.1148/radiol.2020200463.

20. Colombi D, Bodini FC, Petrini M, Maffi G, Morelli N, Milanese G, et al. Well-aerated lung on admitting chest CT to predict adverse outcome in COVID-19 pneumonia. *Radiology.* 2020;296(2):E86–E96.

CHAPTER 6

Using Reactive Machine AI and Dynamic Changes in Lung Structure to Derive Functional Quantitative Lung CT Metrics of COPD, ILD, and Asthma

Introduction

The previous chapter reviewed the lung CT AI methods to assess normal and diseased lung structure using a single TLC chest CT scan. COPD, ILD, and asthma can all produce small and large airway disease. This chapter will look at how lung CT AI can be used to assess lung ventilation by obtaining two chest CT scans with each scan taken at a different lung volume. This approach can be viewed as a dynamic assessment of the lungs that can provide information on lung function by assessing lung ventilation. Functional lung CT imaging can provide indirect information on the function of small airways, <2 mm in diameter, that cannot be measured directly by currently available CT scanners. Direct imaging of the airway tree can provide structural information on normal and diseased airway tree geometry (e.g., lumen area, wall area) at different generations from the trachea, generation 1, to subsegmental airways out to airway generation 6. Direct imaging of the airway tree by chest CT will be discussed later in this chapter.

Expiratory QCT Assessment of Air Trapping Due to Small Airway Disease in the Lung

Obtaining a chest CT scan at a lower lung volume, FRC or RV, can be used to assess air trapping in the lung, areas of the lung where air cannot freely be exhaled. The process of exhaling air out of your lungs decreases the volume of your lung by decreasing the amount of air per unit volume and since the tissue per unit volume is approximately constant, the overall density of the lung tissue normally increases when you exhale (Fig. 6.1). The normal expiratory CT scan obtained at either FRC or RV shows increased density throughout both lungs due to the decrease in air volume in the lung without substantially changing the tissue volume. The lung decreases in size and the density of the lung increases to the extent that air is exhaled from each region of the lungs. This decrease in air is greater in the lower lobes than the upper lobes and is greater in the dependent portions of the lungs compared to the nondependent portions of the lungs (Fig. 6.1).

When there is a narrowing of the small airways in the lung or a reduced number of small airways in the lung or both, the lungs will not exhale as much air as they normally

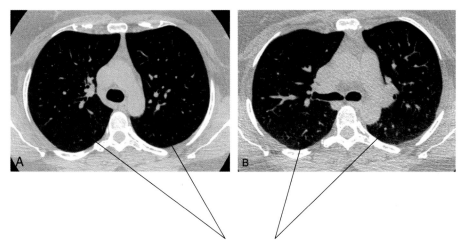

Fig. 6.1 **(A)** Normal supine inspiratory (TLC) chest CT axial image. **(B)** Normal supine expiratory (RV) chest CT axial. Note the increased density in the lungs in **B** due to the decreased air per unit volume of lung. The increase in lung density in **B** is greater in the more dependent portion of both the lungs *(arrows)*. Note the cross-sectional area of both lungs has also decreased in **B**. (Courtesy of VIDA.)

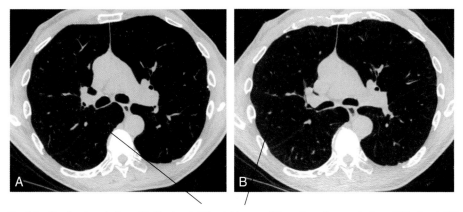

Fig. 6.2 Supine inspiratory (TLC) chest CT axial image **(A)** and supine expiratory (RV) chest CT axial image **(B)** from a patient with severe COPD (GOLD Stage 4). There is little change in lung density throughout both lungs in **B** compared to **A** *(arrows in A and B)*. This lack of change in lung density is due to air trapping from obstruction and/or loss of small airways, <2 mm in diameter (see text). (Courtesy of VIDA.)

would in the regions of the lung where there are abnormal small airways. The areas of lung where there is incomplete emptying of the air will decrease the density of the lung in those regions, compared to the adjacent normal lung tissue, on expiratory chest CT scans. This is referred to as air trapping and is seen on FRC/RV chest CT scans as regions of relative decreased density compared to normal areas of higher density on the expiratory CT scan (Fig. 6.2). The trapped air can be quantitated in several ways and at different scales, including assessing both lungs together, individual lungs, lung lobes, and at the level of the individual lung voxel. Assessing air trapping at progressively smaller scales can increase spatial information that is lost when the air-trapping analysis is done by assessing both lungs together.

The mean lung density on expiration, FRC/RV, CT scans can be used to assess air trapping.[1] Similar to the LAA and HAA measures described in Chapter 5, the amount of lung that is lower than a defined threshold HU value on an FRC/RV lung CT can assess the amount of air trapping in the lung (Fig. 6.3).[2-6] The ratio of the mean lung

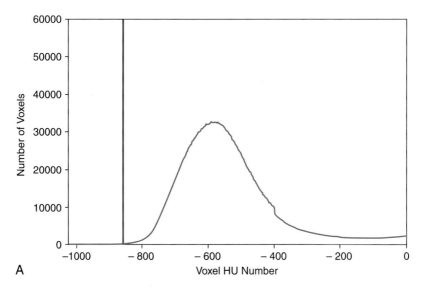

A

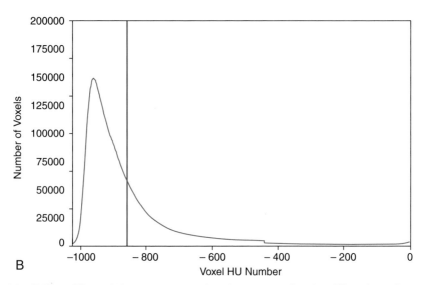

B

Fig. 6.3 RV lung CT voxel histogram curve taken from a normal patient **(A)** and a patient with air trapping from COPD **(B)**. The vertical red lines mark the −856 HU value (**A**, LAA_{-856} = 0.1%, mean lung density (MLD) = −531 HU. **B**, LAA_{-856} = 66.7%, MLD = −854 HU).

BOX 6.1 ■ Qualitative CT Methods to Assess Air Trapping

1. Mean value of the lung CT voxels on an FRC lung CT
   - This is referred to as the expiratory mean lung density ($MLD_{expiration}$)
2. Determine the percentage of FRC or RV lung CT voxels that are <-856 HU
   - This is referred to as the LAA_{-856}
3. Ratio of the FRC lung CT MLD to the TLC lung CT MLD
   - $MLD_{expiration}/MLD_{inspiration}$
4. Ratio of the FRC CT lung volume to the TLC CT lung volume
   - CT_{FRC}/CT_{TLC}
5. Determine the difference between TLC CT lung volume and RV CT lung volume
   - $CT_{TLC}-CT_{RV}$
6. Functional small airway disease using PRM or DPM
   - fSAD

---

density on expiration to the mean lung density on inspiration can also be used to assess the amount of air trapping present in the lung.[7] Air trapping can also be assessed in the lung by taking the ratio of the CT lung volume at FRC to the CT lung volume at TLC.[1] A much more powerful way to assess the air trapping in the lung is to use nonrigid registration methods to compare voxel by voxel the differences in lung attenuation between the TLC and RV chest CT scans. Two well-known published methods that use image registration to assess air trapping at the voxel level: the parametric response map (PRM) and the disease probability map (DPM).[8,9] The different methods to determine air trapping in the lung are summarized in Box 6.1.

WHOLE LUNG ASSESSMENT OF AIR TRAPPING USING LAA IN SEVERE ASTHMA PATIENTS

Air trapping is a hallmark of patients with asthma. Busacker et al. in 2009 reported the results of assessing air trapping in severe asthma subjects enrolled in the Severe Asthma Research Project (SARP) using quantitative assessment of chest CT scans obtained at FRC.[4] Air trapping was defined to be significant in this study if 9.66% or more of the lung tissue was <-850 HU, LAA_{-850}, on the expiratory chest CT scans obtained at FRC. The quantitative chest CT assessment of LAA_{-850} in this study identified severe asthma subjects that were at increased risk for asthma-related hospitalizations, ICU visits, and mechanical ventilation. Multivariate analysis showed that those subjects with an LAA_{-850} $>9.66\%$ had an increased risk of asthma, pneumonia, high levels of airway neutrophils, and airflow obstruction measured by FEV1/FVC ratio and atopy.[4]

WHOLE LUNG ASSESSMENT OF AIR TRAPPING USING LAA IN COPD PATIENTS

Schroeder et al. in 2013 reported the results of doing TLC and FRC quantitative CT scans to assess air trapping and emphysema in 4062 COPD subjects enrolled in the COPDGene research study.[5] The quantitative CT metric of air trapping was defined as the percent or fraction of lung tissue <-856 HU, LAA_{-856}, on the expiratory FRC CT scan (Fig. 6.3). The results of this study showed that the LAA_{-856} metric of air trapping strongly correlated with decreases in airflow measured by spirometry, FEV1 $R = -0.77$ and FEV1/FVC $R = -0.84$, in this large group of COPD subjects. The corresponding LAA_{-950} metric of emphysema derived from the TLC chest CT scans (see Chapter 5) did not correlate as strongly with decreases in airflow, FEV1 $R = -0.67$ and FEV1/FVC $R = -0.76$.

WHOLE LUNG ASSESSMENT OF AIR TRAPPING IN THE COPDGENE 2019 CLASSES OF COPD

As we discussed in Chapter 5, the COPDGene 2019 Classes of COPD are determined by first defining four novel criteria to diagnose COPD: "Exposure, Symptoms, CT Structural Abnormality, Spirometry".[6] The CT structural criteria include having one or more of the following lung CT AI QCT metrics: LAA_{-950} equal to 5% or greater on a TLC chest CT scan (QCT structural measure of Emphysema), $LAA_{-856} \geq 15\%$ on expiratory CT scan (QCT functional measure of air trapping), Pi10 equal to 2.5 mm or greater (QCT structural measure of airway wall thickening).[6] The presence of 15% or more of air trapping on an expiratory FRC CT using the QCT metric LAA−856 in a patient with a 10-pack-year or greater smoking history, means they have at least possible COPD using the COPDGene 2019 Classes of COPD (see Chapter 5).[6]

WHOLE LUNG ASSESSMENT OF AIR TRAPPING USING MLD AND CT DETERMINED LUNG VOLUMES

A recent publication by Pompe et al. reported assessing air trapping in 5697 COPD subjects enrolled in the COPDGene study using the whole-lung mean lung density (MLD_{FRC}) on FRC CT scans and also the ratio of the CT determined lung volume on FRC CT scanning to the CT determined lung volume on the TLC CT $(CT\text{-}FRC_{vol}/CT\text{-}TLC_{vol})$.[1] This study showed significant increases in $(CT\text{-}FRC_{vol}/CT\text{-}TLC_{vol})$ and significant decreases in MLD_{FRC}, both indicators of whole lung air trapping, between baseline TLC and FRC CT scans and 5-year follow-up TLC and FRC CT scans in patients with COPD, GOLD Status 1–4.[1] These results were attenuated but did not resolve when FEV1 was included in the statistical models.[1] The authors indicate that the CT measures of air trapping in patients with COPD can progress without significant change in FEV1. CT determined air trapping are not completely determined by measures of FEV1 and the CT measures of air trapping in this study provide additional information compared to FEV1. The chest CT determined MLD_{FRC} and $CT\text{-}FRC_{vol}/CT\text{-}TLC_{vol}$ are both effective means of assessing air trapping and following the progression of air trapping over time in subjects with COPD.[1]

WHOLE LUNG ASSESSMENT OF AIR TRAPPING IN BRONCHIOLITIS OBLITERANS

Diseases of the small airways, <2 mm in diameter, are referred to as bronchiolitis. there are two predominate forms of bronchiolitis: cellular/proliferative bronchiolitis and obliterative/constrictive bronchiolitis. The primary causes of cellular bronchiolitis are infection, smoking, hypersensitivity pneumonitis, follicular bronchiolitis, and diffuse panbronchi-olitis.[10] The primary causes of bronchiolitis obliterans are postinfection, lung and bone marrow transplantation, connective tissue disease, toxic fume inhalation, adverse drug reactions, and inflammatory bowel disease.[10] Bronchiolitis produces air trapping in the lung, which can be assessed with visual lung CT and lung CT AI methods.

The development of small airway disease in lung transplant recipients has been assessed using lung CT AI.[11] The development of rejection in the transplanted lung can produce narrowing and obstruction of the lumen of small airways. This produces air trapping on expiratory CT scans that can be assessed using QCT metrics of air trapping. The development of small airway disease in lung transplants due to allograft rejection is described as bronchiolitis obliterans syndrome or BOS. Barbosa et al. reported in 2018 their retrospective experience in assessing 178 lung transplant patients who had 3D whole lung TLC and CT scans along with spirometry to assess FEV1, FVC, and FEV1/FVC ratio. Of these patients, 99 had a clinical diagnosis of BOS, and 79 were BOS negative.

The lung CT AI method in this study acquired two high-quality 3D chest CT scans with 1-mm slice thickness obtained at TLC and RV. The lungs on the TLC and RV CT scans were automatically segmented from the rest of the thoracic anatomy. The follow-ing quantitative CT (QCT) metrics were automatically generated for both lungs, indi-vidual lungs, and lung lobes: LAA_{-950} on TLC CT scans, LAA_{-856} on RV CT scans, and lung volume difference between TLC and RV CT scans. Nonrigid registration methods were used to identify the difference in attenuation values (HU) between corresponding voxels at TLC and RV. The number or volume of coregistered voxels that had changed by <75 HU were considered the optimal image registration-driven method for assess-ing air trapping from small airway disease.[11] Whole-lung volume difference (WLVD), left-lung volume difference (LLVD), and right-lung volume difference (RLVD) had the strongest correlations with FEV1.[11]

The study computed the multivariate Pearson correlations of multiple QCT met-rics, as well as multiple visual metrics of BOS on the CT studies. This study showed quantitative CT determined whole lung volume difference (QCT WLVD) between the inspiratory and expiratory CT scans had the strongest correlation with FEV1, in patients who underwent bilateral lung transplants, $R = 0.69$ and $P <0.0001$.[11] The QCT WVLD also had the strongest correlation with FEV1 in patients who had undergone a right lung transplant, $R = 0.69$ and $P <0.0001$, though QCT RLVD was not surpris-ingly very similar, $R - 0.68$ and $P <0.0001$. The QCT LLVD had the highest correlation with FEV1 in patients who underwent a left lung transplant, $R = 0.86$ and $P <0.0001$.[11]

Assessment of Air Trapping at the Voxel Level Using Image Registration

It has been shown that the narrowing and loss of small airways of <2 mm in diameter in COPD subjects is the major site of obstruction to airflow.[12] This loss of small airways is the major cause of air trapping assessed on expiratory chest CT scans. It has also been shown that the loss of terminal bronchioles precedes the development of emphysema in COPD patients.[12] The assessment of air trapping using whole-lung, lung, and lobe expiratory CT scans obtained at FRC or RV in patients who also have emphysema,

---

BOX 6.2 ■ Different Lung Scales Used to Assess Air Trapping

1. Whole lung
   - Both lungs combined
2. Single lung
   - Right and left lung assessed separately
3. Lung lobes
   - Each of the five lung lobes are assessed separately
4. Lung segments
   - Each of the 10 right lung segments and each of the 7 left lung segments are assessed separately
5. Voxel level assessment of air trapping
   - PRM or DPM

---

as is often the case in COPD patients, is an issue, since the areas of emphysema will be included in the air trapping index. The desire to detect air trapping separate from emphysema is to improve the detection of COPD-related lung injury before emphysema develops and to assess treatment effects on air trapping separate from emphysema. This has led to the development of other QCT metrics to assess air trapping apart from whole lung, lung, and lobe assessments. Box 6.2 summarizes the different scales that can be used to assess air trapping.

The issue of assessing air trapping separate from emphysema has led to assessing the lung at the level of the individual chest CT image voxel at different lung volumes (e.g., TLC and FRC/RV). The voxel is the smallest spatial dimension that we can sample in chest CT scans. Fortunately, modern CT scanners can produce images of the lung with isotropic CT, equal in x, y, and z dimensions, and resolution of 0.5 mm. If the lung volume is 5 liters, this corresponds to 40 million voxels. The voxel approach, as opposed to the whole lung approach, to assessing the lungs for air trapping versus emphysema helps in separating the parts of the lung that have air trapping but no emphysema from those areas of the lung with emphysema and air trapping by not averaging the values of the 40 million voxels over the 5-liter lung volume.

The parametric response map (PRM) and disease probability map (DPM) are two voxel-level methods of assessing emphysema, air trapping, normal lung and areas of emptying emphysema, and emphysema and no air trapping present, at the voxel level.[8,9] The individual voxel method handles coexisting emphysema and air trapping in a more robust manner than the lung CT AI methods that assess large groups of voxels (e.g., both lungs together).

PARAMETRIC RESPONSE MAP

Galban et al. in 2013 described a much more sophisticated method of detecting emphysema, as well as air trapping when two chest CT scans were obtained at inspiration, TLC, and expiration, FRC/RV.[8] These investigators used non–rigid image registration methods to coregister each of the voxels in the TLC and FRC chest CT scans on 194 subjects from the COPDGene Phase 1 study. Then each coregistered voxel was assessed for emphysema, voxel value <-950 HU on the TLC scan, and for functional small airway disease, fSAD, voxel value <-856 HU on the FRC chest CT scan. Using this scheme, three uniquely defined groups of coregistered voxels were generated: normal, fSAD, and fSAD + emphysema to form a two-dimensional parametric map of the voxels. This two-dimensional parametric map is called the parametric response map (PRM). In this scheme, if there was no emphysema or air trapping in the coregistered voxel, it was classified as a normal voxel. If there was emphysema and fSAD in the coregistered voxel, it was classified as emphysema, and if there was fSAD and no emphysema in the coregistered voxel, it was classified as air trapping or functional small airway disease (fSAD). This method has subsequently been extended to include a fourth classification of the coregistered voxel where there is emphysema but no fSAD. This is referred to as emptying emphysema. The introduction of nonrigid image registration to assess each paired voxel value change to assess fSAD and fSAD + emphysema was very novel. In this approach, each voxel of the lung can be assessed for the presence of small airway disease, emphysema, or both. The number of pairs of voxels classified as normal, fSAD, fSAD + emphysema, or emphysema can be expressed as a percentage of the total number of voxel pairs to compare with other measures of COPD, including spirometric measures of airflow (e.g., FEV1 and FEV1/FVC).

The assessment of each paired voxel using the Galban method of assessing for fSAD and fSAD + emphysema was reported by Bhatt et al. in 2016.[13] Included in the COPDGene study were 1508 subjects assessed at baseline and a 5-year follow-up with TLC and FRC CT scans, spirometric measurements of postbronchodilator FEV1 and FEV1/FVC, subject demographics, smoking burden, COPD exacerbations, completion of St. George Respiratory Questionnaire, and assessment of dyspnea using the Modified Medical Research Council (mMRC) dyspnea score.[13] This study showed that fSAD, but not fSAD + emphysema, was significantly associated with the decline in airflow measured by FEV1 in smokers without COPD, GOLD 0. The study showed that for every 5% increase in fSAD there was a significant decline in FEV1, 2.2 mL/yr per 5% increase in fSAD. In smokers with COPD, GOLD 1–4, a 5% increase in fSAD produced a significant decline in FEV1, 4.5 mL/yr per 5% increase in fSAD. The fSAD + emphyema metric in smokers with COPD, GOLD 1–4, also showed a significant association with a decline in FEV1, though not as strong as fSAD: 3.5 mL/yr per 5% increase in fSAD + emphysema.[13] This study also showed that fSAD had a stronger association with FEV1 decline than fSAD + emphysema in GOLD 1–4 COPD subjects, and this was the strongest in the GOLD 1–2 subjects. The stronger association of fSAD, compared to fSAD + emphysema in both smokers without and with COPD, supports the concept that has been previously reported, that the narrowing and disappearance of small conducting airways precede the development of emphysema in COPD patients.[12] Lung CT AI using fSAD can detect and assess small airway disease at the voxel scale separate from fSAD + emphysema.

DISEASE PROBABILITY MAP

Kirby et al. in 2017 described an image registration-driven paired voxel method similar to the PRM approach described in *Parametric Response Map* that extended the voxel-based methodology Galban had introduced to improve the detection of air trapping or functional small airway disease.[9] The approach was labeled a disease probability map (DPM).[9] The PRM method uses a fixed threshold of −950 HU to identify emphysema on the TLC CT voxels and a fixed threshold of −856 HU to identify air trapping on the image matched FRC/RV CT voxels.[8] The PRM method classifies voxels into normal, fSAD, fSAD + emphysema, and emphysema without fSAD by using fixed thresholds. Kirby's approach does not use fixed thresholds but instead uses a variable threshold method.[9]

The study by Kirby selected 504 study subjects from the CanCOLD population-based Canadian COPD study. Nonsmokers, smokers without COPD, GOLD 0, and smokers with COPD, GOLD 1–2, were included in the study. Each of the subjects had 3D TLC and 3D RV chest CT scans done using 100 kVp, 50 mAs, 0.5-second x-ray tube rotation time, pitch of 1.375, and a slice thickness between 1.00 mm and 1.25 mm.[9] The TLC and RV chest CT scans used a nonlinear registration algorithm to perform the image matching of the corresponding TLC and RV voxels. Classification of the image-matched voxel pairs were performed by PRM and DPM to classify the paired voxels into normal, fSAD, and fSAD + emphysema.[9] The PRM method used fixed thresholds for detecting fSAD (−856 HU on FRC/RV) and emphysema (−950 HU for TLC) for all the lung voxels. DPM, in contrast, estimates independent probabilities of fSAD and emphysema at each voxel based on the combination of HU value in the TLC scan and the image-matched HU value in the RV or FRC scan. For the assessment of fSAD within the aerated lung, DPM uses the TLC voxel value to assign an exponential decay function whose value is 1.0 (100% fSAD) if there is no difference in the HU value of the paired voxel between TLC and RV. The probability of fSAD decreases exponentially, approaching 0% as the difference in the HU value of the voxel pair increases. For the probability of emphysema, DPM uses an exponential decay function based on the average inspiration and expiration intensity values. The function assigns a probability of 1.0 (100% emphysema) if the average of the inspiration and expiration voxel values is −1000 HU (pure air) and decreases exponentially, approaching 0% as the average inspiration and expiration lung voxel values approach 0 HU. A voxel pair is considered normal if the fSAD and emphysema probabilities are both <0.5 or 50%; fSAD only (no emphysema) if the probability of fSAD is >0.5 or 50%, and the probability of emphysema is <0.5 or 50%; and fSAD + emphysema if both fSAD and emphysema probabilities are >0.5 or 50%.[9]

In Kirby's study, both PRM and DPM correlated equally well with physiologic measures of airflow obstruction (FEV1 and FEV1/FVC) and air trapping (RV/TLC).[9] PRM and DPM were able to identify significant differences in gas trapping between GOLD 2 COPD subjects, at-risk smokers, and never smokers. They were also able to do the same in GOLD 1 subjects compared to at-risk smokers. Only DPM could distinguish GOLD 2 subjects from GOLD 1 subjects.[9]

Assessment of Biomechanics and Tissue Stiffness Using Image Registration

The approach of using image registration in lung CT AI can be extended beyond identifying air trapping and emphysema by using voxel HU values. Using deformable image registration to look at voxel pairs from TLC and FRC/RV chest CT scans can also be used to assess biomechanics or how the lung tissue deforms during respiration. Rather than looking at the change in density between inspiration and expiration of the coregistered voxel, we look at how the voxel volume itself changed between the two lung volumes. The Jacobian determinant is a mathematical method to assess the symmetric expansion or contraction of a structure. Bodduluri et al. in 2017 reported the results of using the Jacobian determinant to assess the deformation properties of the coregistered lung voxels from 490 COPD subjects enrolled in the COPDGene research study.[14] The Jacobian determinant method was compared to the whole lung LAA <-950 HU on the inspiratory chest CT scan (TLC chest CT), a QCT measure of emphysema that we discussed in the previous chapter, along with the whole lung LAA <-856 HU on the expiratory FRC chest CT measure of air trapping which we discussed earlier in this chapter. The whole lung value of the Jacobian determinant was the mean coregistered voxel deformation for the whole lung. The mean whole lung Jacobian determinant was significantly associated with measures of COPD subject symptoms assessed by the St. George Questionnaire, 6-minute walk distance, and BODE index and mortality, independent of the COPD subject's age, sex, race, body mass index, FEV1, smoking history, CT emphysema score, CT air trapping score, airway wall thickness, and CT scanner protocol.[14] The mean Jacobian determinant is a measure of tissue biomechanical elasticity or tissue stiffness. It has potential application in not only the assessment of air trapping and emphysema in COPD patients but could also be applied in patients with stiff lungs from pulmonary fibrosis produced by interstitial lung disease.

Direct Measurements of Large Airway Geometry Using Lung CT AI

The above discussion has been centered on using lung CT AI to assess air trapping to indirectly assess narrowing and/or loss of small airways, diameter <2 mm. Lung CT AI has been used to assess the geometric properties of large airways that can be resolved using 3D chest CT scans. The number of large airways that can be assessed depends on obtaining a high-quality chest CT at TLC. It also depends on specialized airway segmentation software to automatically segment out the airways from the rest of the lung anatomy. These airway trees often need to be further manually edited to ensure the quality of the airway tree.

SEGMENTATION OF THE AIRWAYS OF THE LUNGS

The segmentation of the large airways of the lung requires specialized software.[15–17] The software needs to separate the airways from adjacent arteries and veins within the lung. Fig. 6.4 shows a normal airway tree that has been generated from a high-quality 3D TLC chest CT scan with a slice thickness of <1 mm by using advanced commercial software, VIDA. There is continued research, both in the public and private sectors, to improve the lung CT AI software that automatically, or semiautomatically, extracts the airways, arteries, and veins from a chest CT scan so these structures can be analyzed to extract QCT metrics of normal and disease from airways and vessels in the lung.

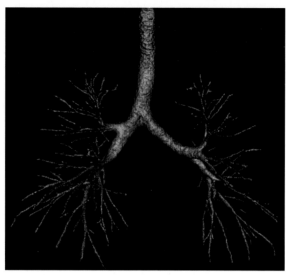

Fig. 6.4   Segmentation of the airways from a normal 3D TLC chest CT using an advanced airway segmentation AI program (VIDA, Coralville, IA). (Courtesy of VIDA.)

QCT METRICS OF AIRWAY GEOMETRY

Nakano et al. in 2000 reported that lung CT AI could be used to extract not only LAA features of emphysema, LAA_{-960}%, but could also extract the geometric features of the apical segmental bronchus of the right upper lobe, RB1, from a group of 94 smokers and 20 asymptomatic volunteers.[18]

Axial scanning mode was used to obtain high-resolution CT (HRCT) images of the lungs using 120 kVp, 200 mA, 1.0-second x-ray tube rotation time. The HRCT images were reconstructed using a DFOV of 320 mm, 512 × 512 reconstruction matrix, and FBP using a Toshiba FC03 kernel. Three HRCT images were used to compute the LAA_{-960}%: one HRCT image 1 cm above the transverse aorta, one HRCT image 1 cm below the tracheal bifurcation, or carina, and one HRCT image 3 cm above the diaphragm.[18] This method of determining LAA_{-960}%, was used for consistency with techniques that had been previously reported in the literature at the time of the study.

3D spiral CT scans were used for the airway analysis. The 3D spiral CT scans were obtained on a Toshiba X-Vigor spiral CT scanner using 120 kVp, 50 mA, and pitch of 1.0. The images were reconstructed using FBP with the Toshiba FC10 kernel, 512 × 512 reconstruction matrix, DFOV of 153 mm to 214 mm targeted to the RUL and RB1, 3-mm slice thickness, and 2-mm slice interval. The following geometric properties of the RB1 airway were extracted automatically by the lung CT AI software: lumen area (Ai), minimum luminal radius termed short radius (SR), maximum luminal radius termed long radius (LR), and wall thickness (T) (Fig. 6.5). The total diameter (D), outer area (Ao), and airway wall area (WA) were derived from Ai, SR, LR, and T. The wall area is shown in Fig. 6.6 represents the difference in area between the outer area (Ao) and lumen area (Ai). The wall area percent was also calculated from WA and Ao, WA/Ao×100. The ratio of the airway wall thickness to total airway diameter ratio (T/D) was also calculated.[18]

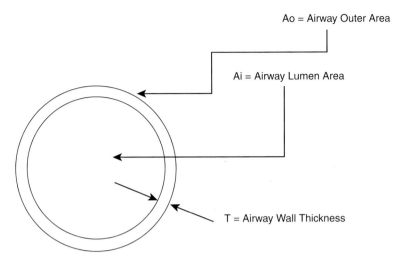

Fig. 6.5 Cross-section of an airway graphically showing the Airway Lumen Area (Ai), Airway Outer Area (Ao), and Airway Wall Thickness (T).

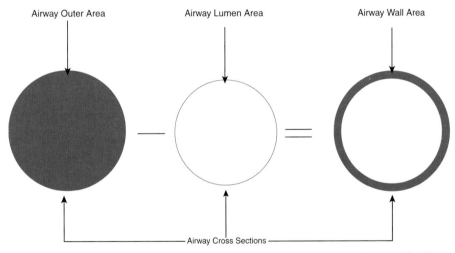

Fig. 6.6 How the Airway Wall Area (WA) is calculated from the Airway Lumen Area and the Airway Outer Area.

The airway metric with the highest univariant regression correlation with the percent predicted FEV1 (FEV1%) was the WA%, $R = -0.338$ and $P <0.001$.[18] The LAA_{-960}% had a higher univariant regression correlation with FEV1% predicted than the WA%, $R = -0.529$ and $P <0.001$.[18] WA% had a stronger univariant significant correlation with FVC%, PEFR%, and RV/TLC% than LAA−960%. LAA−960% had a stronger univariant significant correlation with FEV1%, FEV1/FVC%, and DLCO/VA THAN WA%.[18] Importantly, the inclusion of both WA% and LAA_{-960}% in a multiple stepwise regression analysis showed stronger correlations with FVC%, FEV1%, FEV1/FVC%, PEFR%, RV/TLC%, and DLCO/VA than either WA% or LAA% had in the univariant regression analysis indicating that WA% measures effects that influence pulmonary function that LAA_{-960}% does not capture.[18] The results of Nakano's study suggest the geometric analysis of the segmental airways, conducting airway generation 4, should be pursued in studies of COPD.

COPDGENE AIRWAY GEOMETRY FEATURES AND SPIROMETRIC MEASURES OF AIRFLOW

Schroeder et al. in 2013 reported the results of looking at the segmental airway geometry using lung CT AI in 4542 subjects recruited into Phase 1 of the COPDGene multicenter research study.[5] Each of the subjects in this study had TLC and FRC CT scans. The chest CT scans were obtained on 11 different CT scanner models from three different manufacturers. The number of z-axis detector rows of the MDCT scanners used in the study varied from 16 to 128. The TLC and FRC chest CT scans were obtained using 120 kVp, slice thickness of 0.625 mm, 0.75 mm, and 0.9 mm with corresponding slice intervals of 0.625 mm, 0.5 mm, and 0.45 mm. FBP reconstruction was used to reconstruct the images using a medium or neutral kernel (GE Standard, Phillips B, and Siemens B31f).[5] The TLC CT scans used 200 mAs and the FRC CT scans used 50 mAs. The TLC chest CT scans were used to segment the large airways separately from the rest of the lung CT anatomy.[5] The need for a higher mAs, and hence higher dose to the patients, for the TLC chest CT scan was in part due to the need to have a higher signal-to-noise ratio in the TLC chest CT images so the small structural detail of the large airways could be assessed to the fifth airway generation. The trachea was defined as the first airway generation. The airway tree segmentation was performed using specialized lung CT AI software, Pulmonary Workstation Version 2 from VIDA Diagnostics.[5] Trained research CT image analysts edited the airway trees when necessary. The following airway geometry lung CT AI features were extracted from the fourth-generation airways, segmental airways, and fifth-generation airways: inner area, outer area, inner diameter, inner perimeter, wall thickness, wall area, wall area percentage, and Pi10.[5] The Pi10 is calculated by analyzing all the airways with an inner perimeter between 8 mm and 20 mm, and then performing a linear regression of the inner perimeter versus the square root of the wall area of these airways. The Pi10 is determined from the linear regression analysis by first finding the inner perimeter value of 10 mm on the x-axis and then finding the corresponding square root of the wall area on the y-axis, which is the Pi10 value.

The lung CT airway geometry metrics from fourth-generation/segmental airways had a lower correlation with FEV1, R ranging from 0.15 to −0.44, and FEV1/FVC, R ranging from 0.19 to − 0.34, than LAA_{-950} on TLC CT scans, FEV1 $R = -0.67$ and FEV1/FVC $R = -0.76$, and the LAA_{-856} on FRC CT scans, FEV1 $R = -0.77$ and FEV1/FVC $R = -0.84$. The fourth-generation airway geometry metric with the strongest correlation to FEV1 was WA%, $R = -0.44$. The fourth-generation airway geometry metrics with the strongest correlation to FEV1/FVC were WA%, $R = -0.34$, and inner diameter, $R = 0.34$. A multiple regression model that used the Log10 value of FEV1 as the response variable and LAA_{-950}, LAA_{-856}, fourth-generation airway inner diameter, airway wall thickness, and Pi10 as the explanatory variables showed that by including inner diameter, airway wall thickness, and Pi10 in the model, the correlation improved by 6%, 3%, and 3%, respectively. Similarly, a multiple regression model that used the Log10 value of FEV1/FVC as the response variable and LAA_{-950}, LAA_{-856}, fourth-generation airway inner diameter, airway wall thickness, and Pi10 as the explanatory variables, showed that by including inner diameter and airway wall thickness in the model, the correlation improved by 2.5% and 1.3%, respectively. This study confirms that most of the decrease in FEV1 in COPD subjects is due to loss of elastic recoil measured by LAA_{-950} and small airway disease measured by LAA_{-856}, but lung CT AI metrics of airway geometry (inner diameter, airway wall thickness, Pi10) also can explain part of the decrease in FEV1 in COPD subjects.

PI10 AND COPDGENE 2019 CLASSES OF COPD

As we discussed in Chapter 5, the COPDGene 2019 Classes of COPD are determined by first defining four novel criteria to diagnose COPD: "Exposure, Symptoms, CT Structural Abnormality, Spirometry."[6] The CT structural criteria include having one or more of the following lung CT AI QCT metrics: LAA_{-950} equal to 5% or greater on a TLC chest CT scan (QCT structural measure of emphysema), $LAA_{-856} \geq 15\%$ on expiratory CT scan (QCT functional measure of air trapping), or Pi10 equal to 2.5 mm or greater (QCT structural measure of airway wall thickening).[6] The presence of the lung CT AI airway geometry Pi10 of 2.5 mm or greater on a TLC chest CT in a patient with a 10-pack-year or greater smoking history means they have, in some measure, possible COPD using the COPDGene 2019 Classes of COPD (see Chapter 5).[6] The lung CT AI geometry metric Pi10 will need to be assessed in the future using fully automated systems of lung CT airway segmentation and analysis. This is a big challenge compared to the already very successful lung CT AI lung segmentation software available that is used to compute LAA_{-950} and LAA_{-856}.

Summary

The indirect assessment of small airway disease by assessing air trapping at different scales is a very powerful lung CT AI method to assess patients with obstructive airway disease. The use of image registration to assess air trapping (fSAD) at the voxel level and to assess the Jacobian at the voxel level are very powerful lung CT AI tools to detect and assess a variety of lung diseases that can produce air trapping and increased tissue stiffness. The lung CT AI air trapping metrics that are derived from the segmented 3D lung CT image data in this chapter are computed using reactive AI methods. In the next chapter, we will look at a number of limited memory AI methods to detect and assess diffuse lung disease.

References

1. Pompe E, Strand M, van Rikxoort EM, Hoffman EA, Barr RG, Charbonnier JP, et al. Five-year progression of emphysema and air trapping at CT in smokers with and those without Chronic Obstructive Pulmonary Disease: Results from the COPDGene Study. *Radiology*. 2020. https://doi.org/10.1148/radiol.2020191429.
2. Knudson RJ, Standen JR, Kaltenborn WT, Knudson DE, Rehm K, Habib MP, et al. Expiratory computed tomography for assessment of suspected pulmonary emphysema. *Chest*. 1991;99(6):1357–1366.

3. Newman KB, Lynch DA, Newman LS, Ellegood D, Newell Jr. JD. Quantitative computed tomography detects air trapping due to asthma. *Chest*. 1994;106(1):105–109.
4. Busacker A, Newell Jr. JD, Keefe T, Hoffman EA, Granroth JC, Castro M, et al. A multivariate analysis of risk factors for the air-trapping asthmatic phenotype as measured by quantitative CT analysis. *Chest*. 2009;135(1):48–56.
5. Schroeder JD, McKenzie AS, Zach JA, Wilson CG, Curran-Everett D, Stinson DS, et al. Relationships between airflow obstruction and quantitative CT measurements of emphysema, air trapping, and airways in subjects with and without chronic obstructive pulmonary disease. *Am J Roentgenol*. 2013;201(3):W460–W470.
6. Lowe KE, Regan EA, Anzueto A, Austin E, Austin JHM, Beaty TH, et al. COPDGene® 2019: redefining the diagnosis of chronic obstructive pulmonary disease. *Chronic Obstr Pulm Dis*. 2019;6(5):384–399.
7. Hersh CP, Washko GR, Estepar RS, Lutz S, Friedman PJ, Han MK, et al. Paired inspiratory-expiratory chest CT scans to assess for small airways disease in COPD. *Respir Res*. 2013;14:42.
8. Galban CJ, Han MK, Boes JL, Chughtai KA, Meyer CR, Johnson TD, et al. Computed tomography-based biomarker provides unique signature for diagnosis of COPD phenotypes and disease progression. *Nat Med*. 2012;18(11):1711–1715.
9. Kirby M, Yin Y, Tschirren J, Tan WC, Leipsic J, Hague CJ, et al. A novel method of estimating small airway disease using inspiratory-to-expiratory computed tomography. *Respiration*. 2017;94(4):336–345.
10. Carter BW, Shepard JO, Truong MT, Wu CA. In: Shepard JO, ed. *Thoracic Imaging The Requisits*. Philadelphia, PA: Elsevier; 2019:137–158.
11. Mortani Barbosa Jr EJ, Shou H, Simpsom S, Gee J, Tustison N, Lee JC. Quantitative computed tomography metrics from the transplanted lung can predict forced expiratory volume in the first second after lung transplantation. *J Thorac Imaging*. 2018;33(2):112–123.
12. McDonough JE, Yuan R, Suzuki M, Seyednejad N, Elliott WM, Sanchez PG, et al. Small-airway obstruction and emphysema in chronic obstructive pulmonary disease. *N Engl J Med*. 2011;365(17):1567–1575.
13. Bhatt SP, Soler X, Wang X, Murray S, Anzueto AR, Beaty TH, et al. Association between functional small airway disease and FEV1 decline in chronic obstructive pulmonary disease. *Am J Respir Crit Care Med*. 2016;194(2):178–184.
14. Bodduluri S, Bhatt SP, Hoffman EA, Newell Jr. JD, Martinez CH, Dransfield MT, et al. Biomechanical CT metrics are associated with patient outcomes in COPD. *Thorax*. 2017;72(5):409–414.
15. Palagyi K, Tschirren J, Sonka M. Quantitative analysis of intrathoracic airway trees: methods and validation. *Inf Process Med Imaging*. 2003;18:222–233.
16. Saba OI, Hoffman EA, Reinhardt JM. Maximizing quantitative accuracy of lung airway lumen and wall measures obtained from x-ray CT imaging. *J Appl Physiol*. 2003;95(3):1063–1075.
17. Palagyi K, Tschirren J, Hoffman EA, Sonka M. Quantitative analysis of pulmonary airway tree structures. *Comput Biol Med*. 2006;36(9):974–996.
18. Nakano Y, Muro S, Sakai H, Hirai T, Chin K, Tsukino M, et al. Computed tomographic measurements of airway dimensions and emphysema in smokers. Correlation with lung function. *Am J Respir Crit Care Med*. 2000;162(3 Pt 1):1102–1108.

CHAPTER 7

Using Limited Memory Lung CT AI to Derive Advanced Quantitative CT Lung Metrics of COPD, ILD, and COVID-19 Pneumonia

Introduction

In this chapter, we look at more advanced AI machine learning computer programs for the assessment of normal and diseased lungs using lung CT AI. These AI programs go beyond the reactive machine methods and use the more advanced limited memory AI methods. We have discussed in detail several reactive machine AI approaches to assessing the presence of emphysema, air trapping, and lung fibrosis in Chapters 5 and 6. There is a learning component that precedes the use of reactive machine AI algorithms that select the best analytical lung CT AI metric for a given task. This is seen in the LAA_{-950} in Chapter 5 and LAA_{-856} in Chapter 6. The learning process is done by trial and error, often using linear regression methods, which are a form of machine learning to decide which analytical lung CT metric is best to assess emphysema on a TLC chest CT scan. The −950 HU threshold was "learned" by looking at several thresholds and determining which threshold corresponds best to other independent measures of emphysema (e.g., lung pathology or pulmonary function testing).[1,2]

The process of all lung CT AI methods links together a series of four lung CT AI agents that work together to accomplish a final objective to detect and assess diffuse lung disease (Fig. 7.1). The first step is the CT scanner AI program that generates 3D CT images of the entire thorax. The second step is sending these 3D CT images to a lung segmentation AI program that separates the lungs, airways, and pulmonary vessels from the rest of the thoracic anatomy (e.g., heart, aorta, spine, chest wall muscles). This lung segmentation AI agent is a big enabler in making it possible to analyze a large number of chest CT scans with little or no intervention by human beings.[3] The more advanced lung CT AI lung segmentation software programs use limited memory AI approaches including deep learning. For the third step, the lung segmentation AI program passes the images of the lungs to another AI agent that looks for image features in the lung CT images that can be used to predict certain tissue states (e.g., normal, emphysema, pulmonary fibrosis). The lung features that are extracted by reactive machine AI agents have been described in Chapters 5 and 6. The feature extraction mechanism was hardwired into the reactive memory AI agent without the AI agent needing to learn anything about the lung CT image data. For example, identifying the percent of the lung tissue that was <−950 HU on TLC chest CT scans as a feature of emphysema. The fourth step of lung CT AI is to send the extracted lung CT features to an AI program to detect and

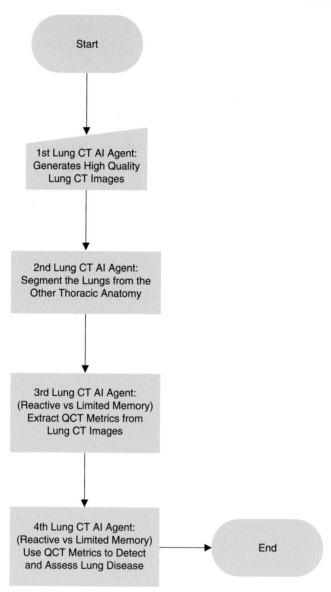

Fig. 7.1 This figure shows a flow diagram of how four lung CT agents work in sequence to detect and assess diffuse lung disease.

assess diffuse lung disease based on the features extracted from the 3D lung CT images. The detection and assessment can be a simple lookup program that assesses if there are any lung CT voxels <-950 HU and, if there are, calculate how many and express this as a percentage of the total lung tissue (e.g., LAA_{-950}) to assess the amount of emphysematous tissue that is present. The LAA_{-950} metric has been previously validated as a viable measure of emphysema, as described in Chapter 5.

In this chapter, we will discuss limited memory (also known as machine learning) lung CT AI agents that train themselves to extract features from the lung CT images that best detect and assess evidence of diseased lung tissue. Supervised training of the limited memory CT AI agent is when the important CT image features are first identified by an expert imaging physician and then the limited memory lung CT agent trains itself to recognize the key features in the image that identify the diseased lung tissue previously identified by the expert imaging physician (Fig. 7.2). The process is unsupervised when the limited memory lung CT AI agent automatically extracts the best imaging features based on the AI agent learning the best lung CT image features to detect and assess the presence of diseased lung tissue (Fig. 7.3).

Supervised training methods of limited memory AI algorithms include support vector machine, decision tree, linear regression, logistic regression, naïve Bayes, k-nearest neighbor, random forest, AdaBoost, and neural network methods.[4] Unsupervised training methods of limited memory AI algorithms include K-means, mean shift, affinity propagation, hierarchical clustering, DBSCAN (density-based spatial clustering of applications with noise), Gaussian mixture modeling, Markov random fields, ISODATA

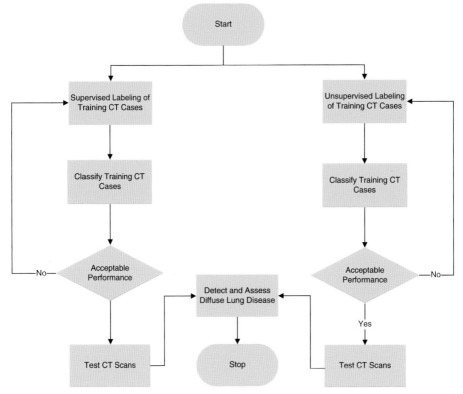

Fig. 7.2 Flow diagram showing the steps both a reactive machine lung CT AI and limited memory lung CT AI program use to detect and assess diffuse lung disease. Either AI approach can use either supervised or unsupervised labeling of CT training cases. The difference in the reactive versus limited memory approach is in how the 3rd and 4th lung CT agents shown in Fig. 7.1 solve the objective of detecting and assessing diffuse lung disease from high-quality lung CT images obtained from the 1st and 2nd lung CT agents also shown in Fig. 7.1.

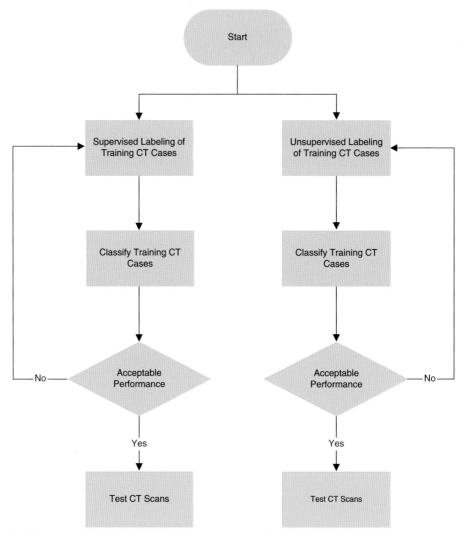

Fig. 7.3 Flow diagram showing the different steps in a limited memory lung CT AI program using either supervised versus unsupervised learning to detect and assess diseased lung tissue.

(iterative self-organizing data), and fuzzy C-means systems.[4] Deep machine learning methods such as convolutional neural networks (CNN) are a recent exciting supervised or unsupervised training method that has been applied recently in the detection and assessment of emphysema and COVID-19 pneumonia;[5] more on this later in the chapter.

After the limited memory lung CT AI agent is trained to detect and assess a class of diseased lung tissue, such as emphysema, pulmonary fibrosis, and pneumonia, it is tested on a new set of chest CT cases that have been labeled by an independent method (e.g., by a human who has visually looked at the CT images for evidence of normal lung tissue, emphysema, pulmonary fibrosis). The results of this testing, or validation step, determine the performance of the supervised or unsupervised machine learning algorithms to detect and quantify important features of lung disease. The results of the AI agent in quantitating the amount of important feature(s) in the CT images, such as emphysema, are often correlated with other measures of disease severity or outcomes (e.g., physiology testing and death rate or mortality).

Limited Memory Lung CT AI and the Assessment of Emphysema

ADAPTIVE MULTIPLE FEATURE METHOD (AMFM) AI AGENT (SUPERVISED, BAYESIAN CLASSIFIER)

The adaptive multiple feature method (AMFM) first described by Uppaluri et al. in 1997 is one of the first lung CT AI papers to use limited memory AI in the assessment of normal and emphysematous lung tissue from chest CT scans.[6] The approach used supervised learning to train the AMFM AI agent. The study had 9 normal subjects and 10 subjects with emphysema. Normal subjects were scanned in the prone position, since they were part of another study looking at interstitial lung disease where prone scanning was done. The emphysematous subjects were scanned in the supine position, since they had advanced COPD and were also being evaluated for lung volume reduction surgery to treat their emphysema. The CT protocol obtained four 3-mm-thick axial images of the lungs obtained using the Imatron Fastrac C-150 XL electron beam CT scanner. Two of the axial CT images were obtained at the level of the carina (tracheal bifurcation), and two were obtained halfway between the carina and the diaphragm.[6]

The different steps that the limited memory AI program AMFM uses are summarized in (Fig. 7.4). The four AMFM steps are in order the following: acquire four 2D lung CT Images, automatically segment the lung tissue from the rest of the thoracic anatomy on the four 2D CT images, expert imaging physician selects regions of interest (ROI) of normal and emphysematous tissue; extract multiple statistical and fractal texture features from training ROI in the four 2D CT images and learn which of these features are optimal for the assessment of normal versus emphysematous lung tissue; detect and assess normal versus emphysema from the test ROI in the four 2D lung CT images based on the prior probability of the extracted features matching normal lung or emphysematous lung.

The third step was accomplished by first having an expert imaging physician label six predefined regions of both the right and left lung on each of the four lung CT images as to whether they were definitely normal or definitely had emphysema. The CT images were then processed so that neighboring voxels of similar values were all assigned an average of the neighboring voxels. These are referred to as the preprocessed ROI. The ROI corresponding to the visually labeled regions of normal and emphysema on the CT images were matched between the unprocessed and processed images. The unprocessed training ROI were then assessed by assessing five first-order statistical features: mean, variance, skewness, kurtosis, grey level entropy, and the geometric fractal dimension. Then the preprocessed training ROI were assessed using eleven second-order statistical features. Five of these second-order statistical features were run-length features and included: short-run emphasis, long-run emphasis, grey level nonuniformity, run-length nonuniformity, and run percentage.[6] The remaining six second-order statistical

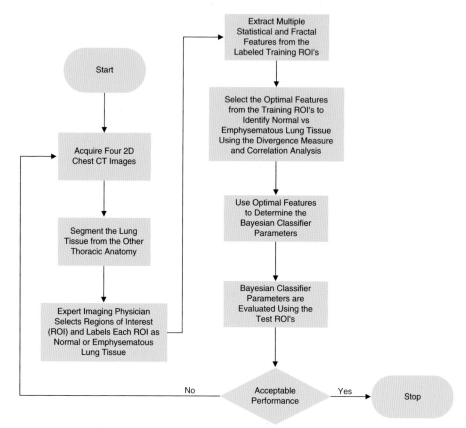

Fig. 7.4 Flow diagram showing the different steps in the AMFM lung CT AI program to detect and assess normal and emphysematous lung tissue, see Adaptive Multiple Feature Method (AMFM) AI Agent (Supervised, Bayesian Classifier).

features were based on the cooccurrence matrix and included: angular second moment, entropy, inertia, contrast, correlation, and inverse difference moment.[6] All of the features were normalized for pixel size and size of the lung in the CT image. The ROI regions that were either definitely normal lung tissue or definitely emphysematous lung tissue were randomly split into two groups of ROI: a training group of ROI used to train the AMFM AI agent and a test set of ROI used to evaluate the ability of the AMFM AI agent to detect normal versus emphysematous ROI. The optimal set of features were selected from the training ROI using the divergence measure along with correlation analysis. Classification into normal and emphysema was done using a Bayesian classifier.[6] The optimal features from the training ROI were used to determine the Bayesian classifier parameters. The ROI from the test set were classified by the Bayesian classifier parameters as to whether the test ROI was normal lung tissue or emphysematous lung tissue. This process could then be repeated to improve the performance/learning of the AMFM lung CT AI agent by adding more labeled normal and emphysematous training and testing ROI. Additional statistical features could also be included to try and improve the performance/learning of the AMFM lung CT AI agent.

The optimal set of features obtained by the AMFM AI agent from the training ROI to separate the normal from emphysematous lung tissue were mean lung density and two run-length features: short-run emphasis and grey level nonuniformity. It is important to note that the mean lung density value of the voxels in the image was an important feature identified by the AMFM AI agent in the training process. Mean lung density is a simple and easy concept to understand that was discussed in Chapter 5. The fundamental lung tissue parameter measured by the CT scans of the lung is lung density. Lung density is known to decrease in patients with emphysema.

The AMFM AI agent was compared to the MLD and the 5th percentile histogram methods for identifying normal versus emphysematous lung. The histogram method looked at the CT number in HU threshold where the lowest 5% of lung voxels occurred. In distinguishing normal lung from emphysematous lung, the AMFM method was 100% accurate, 5th percentile histogram method was 97.4% accurate, and the MLD method was 94.7% accurate.[6] The AMFM AI agent achieved a modest improvement in identifying normal versus emphysematous lung tissue compared to the simpler reactive machine lung CT AI methods in this study.

DEEP LEARNING ENABLES AUTOMATIC CLASSIFICATION OF EMPHYSEMA PATTERN AT CT

Humphries et al. in 2020 reported using a deep learning algorithm that used both CNN and long short-term memory (LSTM) to train a lung CT AI agent to classify patterns of emphysema according to the Fleischner Emphysema Criteria (Fig. 7.5).[7] The Fleischner whitepaper published in 2015 described in detail the visual features of smoking-induced emphysema on chest CT scans.[8] The Fleischner system uses a six-point ordinal scale to visually assess increasing grades of emphysema on chest CT scans. The labels in increasing order of severity are absent, trace, mild, moderate, confluent, and advanced destructive.[8] Between 2007 and 2011, 9652 subjects from the COPDGene study had baseline chest CT scans. These chest CT scans were assessed visually using the Fleischner system. These 9652 subjects also had follow-up mortality information through 2018. A deep learning algorithm was developed using Python Version 3.6 and PyTorch. The input to the convolutional neural network were 25 axial CT images evenly spaced over the z-axis length of the lung, head to toe. The CNN extracted the chest CT image features. The CNN included four blocks with a total of eight layers, four 2D convolutional layers each followed by a pooling layer. The output from the last pooling layer is passed to a concatenation layer that creates a vector of chest CT features that are then passed to a LSTM layer, a kind of artificial neural network, and the output of the LSTM is passed to a dense layer that outputs the probability of each of the six features being present with the total probabilities adding up to 1.0. The final classification score is the probability-weighted average of the categories rounded to the nearest integer.[7]

To train this AI agent, 2407 COPDGene chest CT scans were used. The AI agent was then validated on 7143 separate COPDGene chest CT scans. Additional testing of the AI agent was also done on an additional 1962 subjects from the ECLIPSE research study. The computation time for the AI agent was approximately 60 seconds per chest CT scan. There was moderate agreement in the 7143 COPDGene test chest CT scans between the deep learning emphysema score and the visual emphysema score. The AI agent classified 34% of the cases as one category more severe than the visual score and

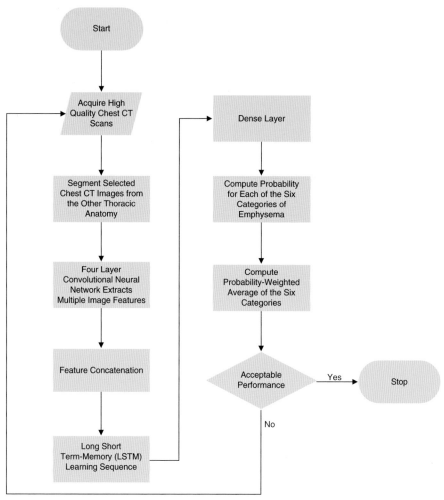

Fig. 7.5 Flow diagram showing the different steps in the limited memory lung CT AI program using a deep learning CNN LSTM method to identify the six increasingly severe forms of smoking-induced emphysema, see Deep Learning Enables Automatic Classification of Emphysema Pattern at CT.

13% of the cases as one category less severe than the visual score. The greatest discordance between the AI agent emphysema score and the visual emphysema score were in those cases where the visual score was normal and the AI agent score indicated trace emphysema.[7] The subjects with normal AI and visual emphysema scores had better measures of airflow (FEV1% predicted and FEV1/FVC ratio) than those subjects with normal visual scores and trace AI agent scores, suggesting the AI agent was detecting real disease with functional significance that the visual score did not. They also had less evidence of emphysema using the less sophisticated AI agent described in Chapter 4 that measures emphysema by determining the amount of lung <−950 HU on TLC CT scans. The AI agent assessment of emphysema severity significantly correlated with the severity of airflow limitation (FEV1 % predicted and FEV1/FVC ratio), 6-minute walk test (6MWT), mMRC dyspnea score (shortness of breath), and the St. George Respiratory Quality (SGRQ) of life score.[7] Similarly, the AI agent emphysema scores were significantly correlated with the clinical stage of COPD. The AI agent emphysema score improved the fit of the visual emphysema score in predicting FEV1 % predicted, FEV1/FVC, 6MWT, and SGRQ of life score adjusting for age, race, sex, height, weight, smoking history, current smoking status, education level, and study site. This indicates that the AI agent emphysema score provides additional information in addition to the visual emphysema score.[7] The AI agent emphysema score predicted increased mortality in subjects with increasing severity scores and the AI agent emphysema score was able to separately predict the mortality risk for Fleischner grade 5 and grade 6 levels, whereas the visual emphysema score could not resolve differences in mortality between grade levels 5 and 6. The AI agent emphysema score predicted increasing mortality as the AI emphysema score increased, even after adjusting for the amount of lung <-950 HU, a simpler AI approach to the assessment of emphysema (see Chapter 4). The training and validation of the CNN AI agent in assessing emphysema was now complete. The CNN AI agent was then tested on a completely separate cohort of 1962 patients. The 1962 patients in the ECLIPSE study had TLC chest CT scans, LAA <-950 HU emphysema score, pulmonary physiology measurements, 6MWT, mMRC dyspnea score, and SGQR score; these were used to test the CNN AI emphysema agent. There were no visual readings done for the ECLIPSE cohort chest CT scans. The CNN AI agent emphysema scores correlated well with increasing severity of FEV1% predicted, FEV1/FVC, 6MWT, mMRC dyspnea score, SGQR score, and increasing LAA <-950 HU scores.[7] This successful testing outcome for the CNN AI agent emphysema severity score suggests that this CNN AI method can be applied to other chest CT scans that are performed to assess smoking-related lung disease to assess the presence and severity of emphysema and predict mortality risk. Tying the CNN AI agent to the visual grades of emphysema established by the Fleischner whitepaper makes it intuitive for the interpreting and treating physicians to understand what the CNN AI agent is doing.[7] The AI agent did better than the visual scoring in the COPDGene validation cohort in assessing physiological impairment, 6MWT, mMRC dyspnea score, and SGRQ quality-of-life score, as well as predicting mortality, suggesting it is capturing additional features of the COPD lung disease that the visual scoring process is not capturing. This could be because there are lung CT features that the human visual process cannot detect.[7]

Limited Memory Lung CT AI and the Assessment of Interstitial Lung Disease (ILD)

AMFM AI METHOD FOR ASSESSING INTERSTITIAL LUNG DISEASE

The AMFM method was described in detail above (**Adaptive Multiple Feature Method (AMFM) AI Agent (Supervised, Bayesian Classifier)**) for its application in assessing normal versus emphysematous lung tissue. The AMFM method has been used to not only assess normal and emphysematous tissue but also to assess ILD due to IPF and Sarcoid.[6,9]

Uppaluri et al. (1999) reported that the AMFM AI method was able to distinguish between normal lung tissue, IPF-related lung disease, sarcoid-related lung disease, and emphysema significantly better than the MLD and Histogram methods.[9] This further supported the notion that the limited memory AI agent approach improved the performance of the reactive machine AI agent approach in identifying and distinguishing between normal and three other different important lung diseases.[9]

CALIPER (COMPUTER-AIDED LUNG INFORMATICS FOR PATHOLOGY EVALUATION AND RATING)

CALIPER is a novel software program implementing an AI agent developed at the Mayo Biomedical Imaging Resource Core that can take chest CT images and, in near real-time, identify features of COPD (emphysema) and ILD (ground-glass opacities (GGO), reticular opacities (RO), and honeycombing (HC)) and quantify the amount of lung that is affected with these features of COPD and ILD (Fig. 7.6).[10,11] The CALIPER AI agent first segments the lungs from the rest of the thoracic anatomy and then segments the airways and pulmonary vessels from the rest of the lung tissue.[10] The CALIPER AI agent uses limited memory AI to learn how to classify different tissue types including normal, emphysema, GGO, RO, and HC. Chest CT scans of

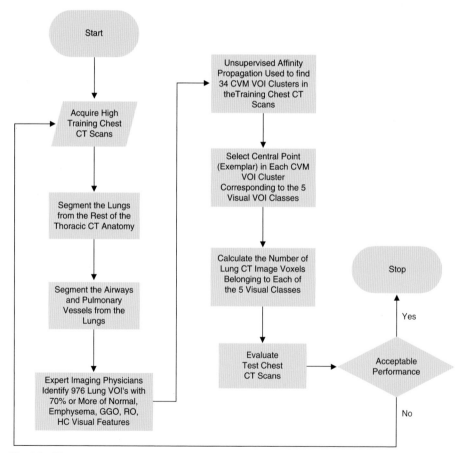

Fig. 7.6 Flow diagram showing the different steps in the limited memory lung CT AI program CALIPER to identify different lung disease tissue types including emphysema, groundglass opacities, reticular opacities, and honeycombing, see CALIPER (Computer-Aided Lung Informatics for Pathology Evaluation and Rating).

14 subjects from the Lung Tissue Research Consortium (LTRC) with the diagnosis of COPD or ILD were used for training the CALIPER AI agent. These 14 chest CT cases were used by expert thoracic imaging physicians to identify 15 mm × 15 mm × 15 mm lung voxel volume of interest (VOI) that were considered to contain 70% or more of the following features: normal, emphysema, GGO, RO, HC. This process identified a total of 976 15 mm × 15 mm × 15 mm VOI: 265 normal VOI, 80 emphysema VOI, 150 GGO VOI, 294 RO VOI, and 187 HC VOI. Pairwise, dissimilarity metrics based on the voxel histograms contained in the same VOI that were visually classified by the expert thoracic imaging physicians were assessed using multidimensional scaling (MDS).[10] The optimal metric was the MDS representation of the Cramer-Von Mises Distance (CVM), which is the L2 metric between cumulative density functions. CVM was the most consistent in matching the VOI voxel values with the visual classification of the VOI.[10] Assessing concordance between the human expert VOI labels (columns) and the unsupervised affinity propagation clustering of the four pairwise CVM dissimilarity metric (rows) of the 976 VOI used to train CALIPER were assessed using the k statistic. K × K tables method (columns × rows) was used to assess the agreement for each visual label.[10] The result of this showed that the CALIPER AI agent grouping of the VOI were well correlated with the visual VOI labels.

The above qualitative agreement of the visual VOI labels with the CVM VOI metric was followed by assessing the quantitative equivalence of the CVM VOI metrics using automatic clustering of CVM similarities. Unsupervised affinity propagation was used to find clusters of CVM VOI in these 14 LTRC training chest CT scans.[10] The unsupervised affinity propagation clustering process identified 34 fundamental clusters and the central point in each cluster, exemplar, that corresponded to the five visual classes of VOI. The number of exemplars for each of the visual features were as follows: nine for normal, five for emphysema, five for GGO, nine for RO, two for normal tissue, and six for HC. This completed the initial training phase of the CALIPER AI agent.

Local 15 mm × 15 mm × 15 mm voxel histograms in the neighborhood of each unknown chest CT lung voxel were compared to the histogram of the 34 exemplars that were identified in the training of the CALIPER AI agent. The CVM dissimilarity measure was calculated between the local voxel histogram and the 34 exemplar voxel histograms identified in the training process and the fundamental type of the exemplar (normal, emphysema, GGO, RO, HC) with the minimum CVM distance was assigned as the parenchymal class of the underlying lung voxel. The number of voxels belonging to normal, emphysema, GGO, RO, and HC were calculated for both lungs and individual lungs. Voxels identified as vessels from the earlier vessel segmentation AI agent were included as normal to account for the total lung volume.

With these results, the CALIPER AI agent also generated a radial space-filling plot, or glyph, that summarized the volume of the five lung lobes and the number or volume of voxels that were classified by the CALIPER AI agent as normal, emphysema, GGO, RO, HC. The glyph, in this report, provides the normal predicted lung volume for the research subject, or patient, by using predictive equations and subject-specific demographics (e.g., age, sex, height, weight) and depicts the normal lung volume using a circular diagram in the glyph.[10,12] The glyph summarized in a very concise geometric diagram the volume of each tissue type the CALIPER AI agent identified in a given chest CT scan of the lungs.[10]

The CALIPER AI agent was tested on the assessment of the lung disease of 119 chest CT scans from patients with known ILD that were taken from the LTRC. These 119 chest CT scans had prior visual assessments and physiologic measurements. The physiologic measurements included forced vital capacity (FVC), diffusion capacity for carbon monoxide (DLCO), and six-minute walk test (6MWT), a measure of exercise capacity. The CALIPER AI agent results significantly correlated well with FVC, DLCO, and 6MWT.[10] The CALIPER AI agent results also correlated significantly with visual assessments of the extent of ILD features including GGO, HC, and RO on these same 119 LTRC ILD cases.[10]

CALIPER has subsequently been used in a number of studies to assess the presence and extent of several interstitial lung diseases, including chronic hypersensitivity pneumonitis, idiopathic pulmonary fibrosis, systemic sclerosis, and rheumatoid arthritis.[11,13–15]

Jacob et al. in 2016 described the use of CALIPER in assessing 283 consecutive patients with idiopathic pulmonary fibrosis (IPF). CALIPER and visual scoring of the chest CT scans on all 283 patients was performed and compared to physiologic measures of lung function, including airflow (FEV1), lung volumes (FVC), and DLCO.[11] CALIPER assessed normal lung, emphysema, GGO, RO, HO, and pulmonary vessel volume (PVV). The CALIPER features were expressed as a percent of the total lung involved with that feature. The CALIPER determined the extent of ILD was the sum of GGO + RO + HO. Visual CT scoring assessed the total extent of ILD to the nearest 5% and subclassified the total score into four features: GGO, RO, HO, and Consolidation. Traction bronchiectasis was given a score of 0 to 3, (none, mild, moderate, severe). The univariate analysis of the relationship of CALIPER determined ILD extent to FEV1 and FVC were superior to the visual assessment of ILD extent. The univariate analysis of ILD extent by CALIPER to DLCO was comparable to visual scoring extent of ILD. CALIPER extent of ILD and PVV had very similar relationships to FEV1, FVC, and DLCO. The PVV value increased with increasing extent of ILD, but this relationship decreased with more advanced cases of IPF.[11]

Jacob et al. in 2017 described the use of CALIPER in the assessment of 116 patients with non-end-stage disease chronic hypersensitivity pneumonitis (CHP). The goal of this paper was to use both visual assessment and CALIPER assessment of chest CT scans of these CHP patients to see what, if any, features predict increased mortality and a poor outcome similar to what one would expect in IPF.[13] The diagnosis of all CHP patients was made in a multidisciplinary ILD conference. Strong univariate predictors of mortality included CALIPER CT assessment of RO, HO, RO + HO (fibrotic score), and PVV, all expressed as a percent of total lung volume. The PVV determined by CALIPER was strongly predictive of mortality in multivariate analysis independent of age, gender, and disease severity. CHP patients with a PVV >6.5% of total lung volume had a mean survival of 35.3 months and a rate of disease progression that closely matched 185 IPF subjects of 38.4 months. PVV was a stronger predictor of mortality than FVC and DLCO in a subanalysis of CHP patients who had histological confirmation of disease or antibody positivity to precipitating antigens after adjusting for age and gender.[13] PVV assessed automatically using the CALIPER limited memory AI agent, was able to predict those CHP patients at high-risk for rapid progression and early death. The PVV is difficult, if not impossible, to assess accurately with a visual approach. CALIPER is providing information that the visual expert cannot not, and in the case of

PVV, this is a real advance in the use of chest CT AI in the assessment of ILD. It is also important to note that in the univariate analysis CALIPER and visual assessment of GGO, RO, and HO were similar in predicting mortality, thus validating the important features the visual observer needs to assess in ILD are also assessed well by CALIPER. Traction bronchiectasis (TxBr) was not assessed by CALIPER but was assessed visually and in univariant analysis, TxBr was a strong predictor of mortality. Interestingly, emphysema assessed both by CALIPER and visually was not predictive of mortality in these CHP patients.

Jacob et al. in 2017 assessed 283 patients with IPF using CALIPER, visual assessment of the chest CT scans, and functional measures of disease (e.g., FVC, DLCO).[16] On multivariate analysis, visual CT parameters of ILD were excluded from the model and the remaining strong independent CT predictors of mortality were CALIPER PVV and CALIPER HO.[16] The study determined that the component of PVV made up of pulmonary vessels >5 mm^2 in cross-sectional area were the most important component vessels in the total PVV score.

Jacob et al. in 2018 published results showing that the CALIPER total vessel-related structure (VRS) score derived from chest CT scans done on a discovery cohort of 247 IPF patients and a validation cohort of 284 IPF patients was able to predict FVC decline at 12 months and survival at 12 months.[17] It was also shown that a CALIPER VRS of >4.4% could be used to enrich a cohort of IPF subjects so that an IPF drug trial sample size could be reduced by 26%.[17]

Jacob et al. in 2019 described the results of using CALIPER, different visual scoring systems (FVC, FEV1, and DLCO) for the assessment of ILD in 157 rheumatoid arthritis (RA) subjects.[15] This study wanted to identify a progressive fibrotic phenotype in rheumatoid arthritis interstitial lung disease (RA-ILD) separate from a less aggressive form of RA-ILD. The study also included 284 subjects with ILD from IPF. IPF is generally a more aggressive form of ILD than RA-ILD but in a subset of RA-ILD patients, RA-ILD is also very aggressive. The univariable analysis of CALIPER assessments of fibrosis (RO + HC), HC, and VRS were powerful predictors of outcome assessed as increases in mortality. The VRS index is used here instead of the PVV metric previously discussed. Using a VRS threshold of ≥4.4% in the multivariable model, RA-ILD subjects had a poorer outcome, similar to the outcome in the IPF subjects. The multivariable analysis results were maintained when the CALIPER extent of ILD or the visual extent of ILD replaced FVC as a measure of baseline disease severity.[15] The mean CALIPER extent of ILD (GGO+RO+HC) was 23.7% in the progressive RA-ILD group and 23.5% in the IPF group. The mean CALIPER VRS was 5.5% in the RA-ILD cohort and 5.3% in the IPF cohort.

DTA (DATA-DRIVEN TEXTURAL ANALYSIS FOR ASSESSMENT OF FIBROTIC LUNG DISEASE)

Humphries et al. in 2017 described a new novel unsupervised limited AI agent that could identify fibrotic lung regions (e.g., combinations of reticular opacities (RO), honeycombing (HO), and traction bronchiectasis (TB)) in patients with interstitial lung disease from IPF (Fig. 7.7).[18] The DTA AI agent was developed by using a training set of 55 3D volumetric CT scans with 1.25-mm-slice thickness or less performed on

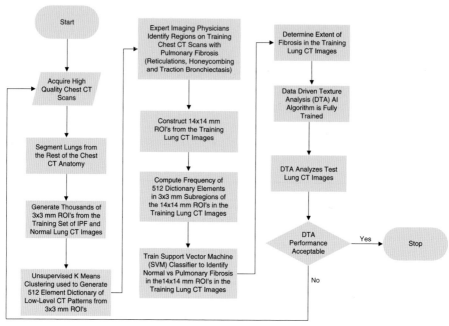

Fig. 7.7 Flow diagram showing the different steps in the limited memory lung CT AI program DTA in the assessment of fibrotic lung disease, see DTA (Data-Driven Textural Analysis for Assessment of Fibrotic Lung Disease).

55 IPF patients. Thousands of 3 mm × 3 mm 2D images were extracted randomly from the 55 training chest CT scans in patients with IPF and from 35 chest CT scans of normal control subjects. A modified k means clustering algorithm was applied to the pixel intensities in these 3 mm × 3 mm images to create a 512 element dictionary of low-level CT image features.[18] Expert thoracic radiologists identified regions of interest (ROI) in the 55 IPF chest CT scans that had RO, HO, and TB or a combination of these features. Training lung CT images, 14 mm × 14 mm ROI, were then constructed. The frequency of occurrence of the 512 dictionary of elements in 3 mm × 3 mm subregions within the 14 mm × 14 mm ROI were then computed. These results were used to train a support vector machine (SVM) classifier to classify 14 mm × 14 mm ROI of lung CT images into either normal lung or fibrotic lung. The DTA determined the extent of fibrosis by dividing the number of 14 mm × 14 mm ROI that were classified as fibrotic and dividing it by the total number of 14 mm × 14 mm ROI in a given chest CT of the lungs. The DTA was used then on 280 validation chest CT cases from subjects with IPF that were not included in the 55 chest CT cases with IPF that were the basis to create the dictionary and train the SVM. The 280 validation CT scans were analyzed using DTA, quantitative histogram measures of fibrosis (see Chapter 5), and visual assessment of the chest CT scans. Each of the 280 validation subjects also had pulmonary function test results of forced vital capacity (FVC) and diffusion capacity for carbon monoxide (DLCO). Seventy-two of these 280 validation chest CT cases also had a follow-up chest CT. The median time between baseline and follow-up CT in these 72 subjects was 14.7 months.

There were significant correlations between baseline DTA fibrotic score, mean lung density, skewness, kurtosis, visual assessment of fibrosis, and baseline values of FVC and DLCO.[18] The quantitative CT metrics correlated better with baseline FVC and DLCO than the visual scoring method. There were significant correlations in the change of the DTA score (lung fibrosis), mean lung density, skewness, kurtosis, and visual assessment of fibrosis, and the change in FVC in the 72 IPF subjects with baseline and follow up chest CT scans and measures of FVC and DLCO. The quantitative measures again outperformed the visual scores. The change in the DTA score, mean lung density, skewness, and visual score significantly correlated with the change in DLCO. The change in DTA score and visual score outperformed the change in mean lung density and skewness in assessing the change in DLCO from baseline to follow-up.[18]

CNN for COVID-19 Pneumonia

The COVID-19 pandemic caused by the severe acute respiratory syndrome coronavirus 2 (SARS-CoV-2) affecting the entire world is still ongoing at the time of this writing, December 2021. The typical COVID-19 viral pneumonia appearance on chest CT scans is that of bilateral, lower lobe, peripheral ground–glass, and consolidative opacities.[19] The peripheral ground-glass opacities may be rounded in appearance and the presence of intralobular septal thickening have been noted in the areas of ground-glass opacity with crazy-paving pattern.[19] Linear opacities and reversed halo sign have been observed as well. There is also a propensity for the ground-glass and consolidative opacities to involve the dorsal or posterior region of the lung lobes. When the typical appearance of COVID-19 pneumonia is present, the diagnosis should be suspected, however, there is an indeterminant pattern of COVID-19 pneumonia on chest CT that overlaps other forms of infectious pneumonia and noninfectious diseases of the lung.[20] The observation that the visual appearance of COVID-19 pneumonia has a recognizable pattern inspired deep learning research to develop an AI agent to recognize COVID-19 pneumonia separate from other infectious pneumonia and other lung diseases.

Li et al. in 2020 reported using a deep learning model entitled COVID-19 detection neural network (COVNet) that extracted the visual features of volumetric chest CT scans for the detection of COVID-19 viral pneumonia separate from other community-acquired pneumonia (CAP) and other noninfectious lung diseases, COPD for example, as well as separate from normal chest CT studies (Fig. 7.8).[5] The chest CT scans used for training the deep learning algorithm included 400 patients with COVID-19 pneumonia, 1396 with CAP, and 1173 without infectious pneumonia. The independent chest CT scans used to test the deep learning algorithm included 68 COVID-19 patients, 155 CAP patients, and 130 without infectious pneumonia. All of the COVID-19 patients that were included in the study had positive RT-PCR tests that confirmed the diagnosis of acute COVID-19 viral pneumonia.

The lungs were first segmented from the rest of the 3D chest CT anatomy using a U-net based segmentation method. The lung CT images were then input into the COVNet framework that consists of a ResNet50 backbone which extracts the features from the lung CT images and then these are combined in a max-pooling operation. The final feature map is fed to a fully connected layer and a softmax activation function is used to generate a probability score for each category, or class, of patients, COVID-19,

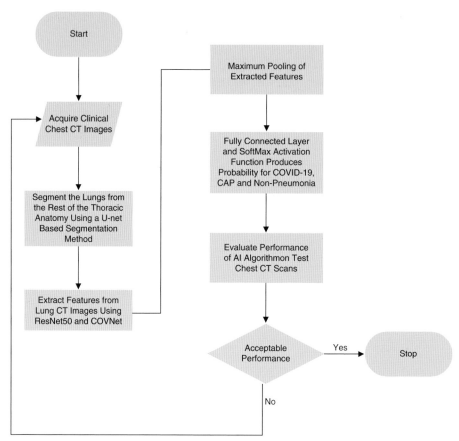

Fig. 7.8 Flow diagram showing the different steps in the limited memory lung CT AI program COVNet in assessing COVID-19 viral pneumonia from other infectious and noninfectious lung disease, see CNN for COVID-19 Pneumonia.

CAP, or noninfectious.[5] The average processing time for the deep learning COVID-19 model was 4.51 seconds using a 3.5 GHz CPU (Intel Xeon Processor E5-1620v4), 16 GB of RAM, and a GPU (NVIDIA Quadro M4000 8 GB). The sensitivity and specificity of the AI COVID-19 agent to detect COVID-19 viral pneumonia on the independent testing set of chest CT studies was 90% and 96%, respectively.[5] The sensitivity and specificity of the COVNet AI agent to detect CAP on the independent testing set of chest CT studies were 87% and 92%, respectively. The area under the ROC curve (AUC) from the independent testing set for COVID-19 pneumonia was 0.96 and for CAP was 0.95. The AUC (area under the ROC curve) is expressed from 0 to 1.0. An AI model whose predictions are 100% correct has an AUC of 1.0. An AI model whose predictions are 100% wrong has an AUC of 0.0. The sensitivity and specificity of the COVNet AI agent to detect nonpneumonia were 94% and 96%, respectively, with an AUC of 0.98.

At the time of this writing, December 2021, the COVID-19 pandemic has seen the publication of many CT AI lung imaging papers. Deng and Li recently reviewed the

COVID-19 AI lung imaging literature.[21] They included 96 papers in this review that were published between January 1, 2020 and March 31, 2021. This review included x-ray projection radiography and x-ray computed tomography of the lungs. The authors discuss AI lung image segmentation methods, AI lung imaging performance in the detection and diagnosis of COVID-19 pneumonia, and AI lung imaging results in the assessment of COVID-19 pneumonia severity and predicting patient prognosis. The authors also provide information on where to access anonymized lung imaging datasets from patients with COVID-19 pneumonia.[21] The authors point out that currently, it is hard to compare the performance of the different AI machine learning methods. This is because the different machine learning methods are developed using different lung imaging datasets to train and validate the AI models and also use different metrics to assess the performance of the models. AI machine learning requires large amounts of quality image data with quality image annotations. This is especially a problem for deep learning methods like the one described above by Li. There is also concern that the lung imaging data is biased toward critically ill patients with life-threatening pneumonia and not enough lung imaging data from patients with less severe pulmonary infections or other lung diseases. There also needs to be more robust AI methods to combine the lung imaging data with other nonimaging data, such as age, blood tests, and RT-PCR tests for COVID-19. AI Deep learning models of lung CT imaging data that predict a given patient has COVID-19 pneumonia suffer from limitations in explaining what structures in the lung are the basis of this decision.[21]

Summary

The limited memory AI programs described in this chapter for the assessment of COPD-related emphysema, ILD-related pulmonary fibrosis, and COVID-19 viral pneumonia are impressive. They are significantly more complex than the reactive AI programs discussed in Chapters 5 and 6. The additional complexity of limited memory AI promises more impressive results than the reactive AI methods if large quantities of unbiased high-quality CT lung image data are available for training, validation, and testing of the AI limited memory AI methods.

Chapter 8 will look at how the anatomic and functional features of the lung that are captured by lung CT AI can be used to build software models of human lung structure and function, and how these software models of the lung can make powerful predictions regarding an individual patient's lung ventilation and perfusion.

References

1. Gevenois PA, de Maertelaer V, De Vuyst P, Zanen J, Yernault JC. Comparison of computed density and macroscopic morphometry in pulmonary emphysema. *Am J Respir Crit Care Med*. 1995;152(2):653–657.
2. Gevenois PA, De Vuyst P, de Maertelaer V, Zanen J, Jacobovitz D, Cosio MG, et al. Comparison of computed density and microscopic morphometry in pulmonary emphysema. *Am J Respir Crit Care Med*. 1996;154(1):187–192.
3. Mansoor A, Bagci U, Foster B, Xu Z, Papadakis GZ, Folio LR, et al. Segmentation and image analysis of abnormal lungs at CT: current approaches, challenges, and future trends. *Radiographics*. 2015;35(4):1056–1076.

4. Erickson BJ, Korfiatis P, Akkus Z, Kline TL. Machine learning for medical imaging. *Radiographics.* 2017;37(2):505–515.

5. Li L, Qin L, Xu Z, Yin Y, Wang X, Kong B, et al. Artificial intelligence iistinguishes COVID-19 from community acquired pneumonia on chest CT. *Radiology.* 2020. https://doi.org/10.1148/radiol.2020200905.

6. Uppaluri R, Mitsa T, Sonka M, Hoffman EA, McLennan G. Quantification of pulmonary emphysema from lung computed tomography images. *Am J Respir Crit Care Med.* 1997;156(1):248–254.

7. Humphries SM, Notary AM, Centeno JP, Strand MJ, Crapo JD, Silverman EK, et al. Deep learning enables automatic classification of emphysema pattern at CT. *Radiology.* 2020;294(2):434–444.

8. Lynch DA, Austin JH, Hogg JC, Grenier PA, Kauczor HU, Bankier AA, et al. CT-definable subtypes of chronic obstructive pulmonary disease: A statement of the Fleischner Society. *Radiology.* 2015;277(1):192–205.

9. Uppaluri R, Hoffman EA, Sonka M, Hunninghake GW, McLennan G. Interstitial lung disease: a quantitative study using the adaptive multiple feature method. *Am J Respir Crit Care Med.* 1999;159(2):519–525.

10. Bartholmai BJ, Raghunath S, Karwoski RA, Moua T, Rajagopalan S, Maldonado F, et al. Quantitative computed tomography imaging of interstitial lung diseases. *J Thorac Imaging.* 2013;28(5):298–307.

11. Jacob J, Bartholmai BJ, Rajagopalan S, Kokosi M, Nair A, Karwoski R, et al. Automated quantitative computed tomography versus visual computed tomography scoring in idiopathic pulmonary fibrosis: validation against pulmonary function. *J Thorac Imaging.* 2016;31(5):304–311.

12. Crapo RO, Morris AH, Gardner RM. Reference spirometric values using techniques and equipment that meet ATS recommendations. *Am Rev Respir Dis.* 1981;123(6):659–664.

13. Jacob J, Bartholmai BJ, Egashira R, Brun AL, Rajagopalan S, Karwoski R, et al. Chronic hypersensitivity pneumonitis: identification of key prognostic determinants using automated CT analysis. *BMC Pulm Med.* 2017;17(1):81.

14. Ferrazza AM, Gigante A, Gasperini ML, Ammendola RM, Paone G, Carbone I, et al. Assessment of interstitial lung disease in systemic sclerosis using the quantitative CT algorithm CALIPER. *Clin Rheumatol.* 2020. https://doi.org/10.1007/s10067-020-04938-3.

15. Jacob J, Hirani N, van Moorsel CHM, Rajagopalan S, Murchison JT, van Es HW, et al. Predicting outcomes in rheumatoid arthritis related interstitial lung disease. *Eur Respir J.* 2019;53(1).

16. Jacob J, Bartholmai BJ, Rajagopalan S, Kokosi M, Nair A, Karwoski R, et al. Mortality prediction in idiopathic pulmonary fibrosis: evaluation of computer-based CT analysis with conventional severity measures. *Eur Respir J.* 2017;49(1).

17. Jacob J, Bartholmai BJ, Rajagopalan S, van Moorsel CHM, van Es HW, van Beek FT, et al. Predicting outcomes in idiopathic pulmonary fibrosis using automated computed tomographic analysis. *Am J Respir Crit Care Med.* 2018;198(6):767–776.

18. Humphries SM, Yagihashi K, Huckleberry J, Rho BH, Schroeder JD, Strand M, et al. Idiopathic pulmonary fibrosis: data-driven textural analysis of extent of fibrosis at baseline and 15-month follow-up. *Radiology.* 2017;285(1):270–278.

19. Bernheim A, Mei X, Huang M, Yang Y, Fayad ZA, Zhang N, et al. Chest CT findings in Coronavirus Disease-19 (COVID-19): relationship to duration of infection. *Radiology.* 2020. https://doi.org/10.1148/radiol.2020200463.

20. Simpson S, Kay FU, Abbara S, Bhalla S, Chung JH, Chung M, et al. Radiological Society of North America expert consensus statement on reporting chest CT findings related to COVID-19: endorsed by the Society of Thoracic Radiology, the American College of Radiology, and RSNA. *J Thorac Imaging.* 2020. https://doi.org/10.1148/ryct.2020200152.

21. Deng H, Li X. AI-empowered computational examination of chest imaging for COVID-19 treatment: a review. *Front Artif Intell.* 2021;4:612914.

Lung CT AI Enables Advanced Computer Modeling of Lung Physiome Structure and Function

Virtual Physiological Human and a Lung Physiome Model

The International Union of Physiological Physiome project was the foundation for the Virtual Physiological Human (VPH) initiative and the human physiome.[1,2] The term *physiome* describes the physiology of the whole organism.[3]

The concept of computational physiology and the human physiome is to have mathematicians and bioengineers, working together with physiologists and molecular biologists, link together the different scales of human biology quantitative models beginning with genomic and proteomic databases, and linking these to higher levels of organization at the cell, tissue, organ, and whole organism level.[2] The mathematical and engineering tools needed to develop quantitative models of physiological dynamics and functional behavior of the intact organism need to account for inhomogeneous, anisotropic, and nonlinear behavior of biological materials.[2]

A complete computational model of lung function will need to span multiple spatial and temporal scales (multiscale model). This is necessary to understand how dynamic molecular interactions at small spatial dimensions link to whole lung function at large spatial dimensions. A multiscale model will use a computationally efficient strategy to capture the important functions for each spatial and temporal scale.[1,4]

Physical forces acting on the surface of the lung through coupling with the chest wall are transmitted to the level of the gas exchange tissue, pulmonary acinus, where this force holds the blood vessels and airways open. The lung surface forces are further transmitted to the level of cells and molecules within the lung tissue where the local stress produced by the lung surface force modulates local cellular and molecular functions.[4]

The stretching of lung tissue produces secretion of surfactant from the type II alveolar epithelial cells that line the pulmonary acinus along with the type I alveolar epithelial cells. The release of surfactant reduces the surface tension of the air-tissue surface of the pulmonary acinus, which decreases the lung surface forces needed to keep the acinar lumen from collapsing and, in this way, alters global lung mechanics.[4]

Pulmonary airway antagonists, such as inhaled allergens (e.g., pollen), act at the cellular level by inducing airway smooth muscle contraction. This results in a subsequent larger-scale narrowing of airway lumens. The narrowed airway lumens in turn produce increases in airway resistance. The increase in airway resistance then produces an even larger scale decrease in whole lung ventilation.[4]

The obstruction of a pulmonary artery lumen by acute thromboemboli, blood clot, induces local disruption of pulmonary artery blood flow that alters the shear stress of endothelial cells on a small scale in the area of the blood clot where pulmonary blood flow has decreased. This decrease in shear stress on the endothelial cells activates the release of nitric oxide by the endothelium, which is a potent vasodilator. The nitric oxide dilates on a larger scale the pulmonary vessels. The dilation of the pulmonary vessels alters on an even larger scale whole lung blood flow.[4]

This chapter will discuss a sophisticated human lung physiome model that includes patient-specific 3D lung CT images as the structural input to a patient-specific multiscale lung model that predicts whole lung physiology of the patient.[1,4–8] In previous chapters we have seen how different lung CT AI can assess lung density for the presence of emphysema and pulmonary fibrosis. We have discussed how combining information from inspiratory and expiratory chest CT scans can be used to assess ventilation at different scales in the lung (e.g., whole lung, lobe, voxel). We have also seen how powerful limited memory AI algorithms can be used to detect and assess different texture patterns produced by diffuse lung disease and to assess whether a lung nodule is benign or malignant. In this chapter, we will see how the 3D lung CT structure of the lung including airways, pulmonary arteries, and veins can be used to construct a patient-specific multiscale finite element model of the lung that can predict hypoxemic risk due to acute pulmonary emboli.[1,4,9]

Tawhai et al. published details of their lung physiome/VPH model.[1,4–10] We will refer to this model as the LP model in this chapter. The LP model builds a complete model of lung structure and how this structure interacts with lung function across a wide range of spatial scales, physical functions, and their integration.[1] The robustness of the LP model is applicable to a wide range of physiological and pathophysiological areas of interest.

The LP model is applicable not only to the risk of gas exchange impairment elevating right ventricular pressure in patients with acute pulmonary embolism but also to the mechanics of airway hyperresponsiveness at the scale of airway smooth muscle to the scale of whole lungs.[1] The LP model can also assess the effects of normal aging on tissue mechanics and optimize methods of mechanical ventilation of the lungs.[1]

Finite Element Model of Lung Structure and Function

There are several major steps in building the LP model of the lung.[4] High-quality 3D chest CT scan is acquired of the thorax and the lungs are segmented from the rest of the thoracic anatomy. The airway tree and pulmonary arteries and veins are segmented from the lung CT images. A 3D finite element mesh of the lungs is generated and bounded by the 3D lung CT volume. The airways are placed into the 3D finite element model and attached to the 3D finite element mesh of the lungs. The extra-acinar and intra-acinar pulmonary arteries and veins are placed into the model. The model then computes known biophysical properties of the lung and includes them in the LP model (Box 8.1).

GENERATING THE 3D FINITE ELEMENT MESH OF THE LUNG

The method of developing a finite element model of the lung begins by geometrically fitting a volumetric finite element mesh, tetrahedrons, or some other 3D polygon, to the

---

BOX 8.1 ■ Steps to Build Patient-Specific Lung Physiome (LP) Model

1. Acquire high-quality 3D chest CT scans of the thorax and segment the lungs from the rest of the thoracic anatomy
2. Segment the airway tree and pulmonary arteries and veins from the lung CT images
3. Generate a 3D finite element mesh of the lungs that is bounded by the 3D lung CT volume
4. Place the airway tree into the 3D finite element mesh of the lung and attach the airway tree to the 3D finite element mesh
5. Place the extra-acinar pulmonary arteries and veins into the 3D finite element mesh
6. Place the intra-acinar pulmonary arteries and veins into the 3D finite element mesh
7. Compute known biophysical properties of the lung and include them in the LP model

---

3D volume of the lungs obtained from a 3D lung CT scan.[4] The volume mesh is then filled with a grid of uniformly spaced points with each point representing a pulmonary acinus; recall there are about 32,000 pulmonary acini in an adult lung. The acinus grid is uniformly spaced assuming that the lung tissue is uniformly expanded at total lung capacity (TLC). This is a reasonable assumption for an upright human lung where maximal expansion can be attained, however, this is less likely in a supine human lung.

GENERATING THE AIRWAY TREE WITHIN THE 3D MESH OF THE LUNG

An initial 1D finite element mesh is placed along the centerlines of the segmented airways obtained from a 3D chest CT scan and acts as an initial condition for the algorithm.[4] Additional new 1D airway branches are generated at the end of a previous branch by directing a branch toward the center of mass of a subset of the acinus grid points where points in any current subset are those that are closest to the parent branch. This process continues until each acinus grid point is supplied by a single terminal model airway.[4] This models the actual lung anatomy where the terminal bronchiole, approximately airway generation 16, supplies a single lung acinus. Tawhai's finite element lung model generates a subject-specific airway tree for the larger airways that are visible on the 3D lung CT and a shape constraint of the subject-specific airway tree using the surface of the 3D lung CT.[4] The algorithmically generated airways cannot exactly match the individual's airway tree beyond those identified by the 3D lung CT; however, the averaged airway geometry of the model is consistent with measured human airway morphometry. Because the anatomically structured airway model is generated within the volumetric finite element model of the lung, the modeled airways are connected to the volumetric finite element model of the lung, and as the lung deforms, so will the airways. This coupling of airway and lung tissue function is a strength of Tawhai's finite element lung model.

GENERATING THE PULMONARY VASCULAR TREE

Modeling tractable, anatomy-based, computationally functional models of the pulmonary vasculature that capture the important structural features of the pulmonary circulation is a big challenge. Each of the dichotomously branching bronchial airways is accompanied by a corresponding dichotomously branching pulmonary artery, but there are many more pulmonary artery branches in the lung than there are airway branches.[4] The additional pulmonary arteries that do not accompany an airway and pulmonary veins are referred to as *pulmonary supernumerary vessels*, and these do not branch dichotomously.[4] The extra-acinar and intra-acinar pulmonary blood vessels have distinct geometric structures that give rise to scale-specific functions.[4] The extraacinar dichotomously branching pulmonary arteries supply blood to the gas exchange units, pulmonary acini, in a parallel arrangement.[4] The intraacinar vascular structure has both series and parallel perfusion. The extraacinar and intraacinar blood vessels need to be modeled differently.[4]

Modeling the Extra-Acinar Pulmonary Vessels

The extra-acinar blood vessels were modeled by Burrowes et al. by constructing models of the extra-acinar blood vessels, including supernumerary vessels, using the 3D lung CT to segment the largest pulmonary vessels and then using a volume filling algorithm, similar to the airway model previously described (See "Generating the Airway Tree Within the 3D Mesh of the Lung" section), to construct the blood vessels accompanying the airways to the level of the terminal bronchiole.[1,4,9] The supernumerary vessels were constructed in a postprocessing step using an algorithm designed to mimic the limited known features of supernumerary vessels. The algorithm assumes the supernumerary vessels have a branch angle close to 90 degrees from the parent vessel and bifurcate rapidly to supply the closest lung parenchymal tissue. The blood vessels are represented as 1D finite elements distributed in the 3D finite element model of lung tissue.

Modeling the Intra-Acinar Pulmonary Vessels

Clark has modeled the intra-acinar blood vessels separately from the extra-acinar blood vessels described above (See "Generating the Airway Tree Within the 3D Mesh of the Lung" section).[11] This model of intra-acinar blood flow separates the small arterioles and venules from the capillary vessels of the acinus. The acinar arterioles and venules are represented as distinct elastic vessels following the branching structure of the acinar airways, respiratory bronchioles, and alveolar ducts. These acinar arterioles and venules are assumed to join each other at each intra-acinar airway generation by a capillary sheet that covers the alveoli present at each generation of acinar airways forming a ladderlike structure. This model accounts for both serial and parallel perfusion pathways in the pulmonary acinus so it can reproduce the decrease in blood flow rates in the distal part of the acinus compared to the proximal part. The ladderlike model of the intra-acinar vessels is novel.[4,11] When the ladderlike model of intra-acinar blood vessels was connected to a symmetric extra-acinar vascular structure, a decrease in pulmonary vascular resistance was observed, compared to a different intra-acinar blood vessel model where each acinus was represented by a single continuous capillary sheet (e.g., only parallel perfusion).

Lung Physiome (LP) Model Applied to the Assessment of Acute Pulmonary Embolism

CT pulmonary angiography (CTPA) is the imaging modality of choice for assessing patients suspected to have acute pulmonary embolism (APE).[12] CTPA is widely available in emergency rooms and hospitals for the assessment of APE. CTPA requires the intravenous injection of iodinated contrast media and is more invasive than the other lung CT methods we have discussed. CTPA has the advantage that it can be performed rapidly and interpreted rapidly by expert imaging physicians. It has largely replaced nuclear scintigraphy for the assessment of acute pulmonary emboli.[12] The identification of acute pulmonary arterial thromboemboli is straightforward; however, the correlation of the size and number of pulmonary emboli does not provide a complete assessment of hypoxemic risk in a given patient with APE.[1]

The LP model is a flexible and reducible model that uses a 3D lung CT to inform a structure-based approach to understand individual patient structure-function interactions. The LP model applied to APE has been helpful in the risk stratification of patients with APE and performs better than the simpler 3D lung CT approach of assessing APE by simply assessing the amount of intravascular clot in the pulmonary arteries.[1] The clot burden, or load, is an example of a "structure"-only approach. There is considerable variation in the severity of APE and patient outcomes in APE who have the same clot burden.[1] The success of the LP model in APE is a good example of how powerful lung physiome models like LP can form the respiratory component of a "virtual patient model (VPM)".[1,10]

The LP patient-specific model used to assess APE utilized contrast-enhanced 3D lung CT tailored to the assessment of the pulmonary arteries (CTPA) and patient demographics; data of patients who were being clinically assessed for possible APE at the Auckland City Hospital, Auckland, New Zealand.[1,5,9]

The 3D distribution of the pulmonary emboli, blood clots, was a semiautomated process that was validated against visual lung CT assessment of the locations of the clots within both lungs.[1] Each clot was associated with a pulmonary artery, and the degree of obstruction depended on the clot size. The LP model then simulated each subject lung perfusion, lung ventilation, and lung oxygen transfer to assess the "hypoxemic risk" for each patient.[1,5,9]

Lung perfusion was modeled using a steady-state blood flow model that assumes Poiseuille flow in the elastic extracapillary pulmonary arterial vessels.[1,4,9] The lung perfusion model uses a "ladderlike" model of the intra-acinar blood flow in each acinus.[11] This perfusion model was embedded within an upright elastic model of the lung parenchyma where each pulmonary vessel and intra-acinar capillary sheet was attached to points in the elastic lung model so that each vessel and capillary sheet responds to the local tethering force transmitted through the upright elastic model attachment points. This local tethering force is a function of the 3D position in the lung and lung posture (e.g., upright versus supine).[1] The inclusion in the perfusion model of intra-acinar structure and function allowed the LP model to redistribute blood flow from the area of lung that had occluded pulmonary arteries from APE to other regions of the lung without blood clots.[1]

Lung ventilation was simulated using a quasi-steady-state model of 1D airflow that included energy loss equations in the conducting airways, generations 116, that were subtended by compliant pulmonary acinar tissue units.[1] An equation of motion was calculated to balance the elastic tissue pressure, terminal bronchiole air pressure, and airflow.[1]

Oxygen gas transfer from the air contained within the acinar lumen to the blood in the capillary sheet of the acinar unit was modeled assuming equilibration of oxygen

> **BOX 8.2** ■ **Boundary Condition Parameters for the LP Perfusion and LP Ventilation Models**
>
> 1. Heart rate (BMP) = 65 beats per minute
> 2. Cardiac output
> 3. Left arterial pressure
> 4. Metabolic rate
> 5. Oxygen uptake
> 6. Respiratory rate (RR) = 12 breaths per minute
> 7. Minute ventilation (tidal breathing)

between the air containing acinar lumen and the blood, containing lumen of the capillary within the capillary sheet. The patient was assumed to be hemodynamically stable, having stable blood pressure and pulse.[1] The Kapitan and Hempleman model was used to calculate the steady-state partial pressures of oxygen (O_2) and carbon dioxide (CO_2) in each acinus.[1] The partial pressures of O_2 and CO_2 within the gas-containing portion of the pulmonary acinus were calculated assuming the steady-state condition and were set equal to their values of the partial pressures of O_2 and CO_2 within the blood containing lumen at the end of each capillary of the acinar capillary sheet. The pulmonary venous partial pressure of O_2 and CO_2 were calculated averages of end-capillary O_2 and CO_2 contents that were then converted to partial pressures of O_2 and CO_2.[1]

The LP perfusion model needed specific boundary conditions set for cardiac output and left atrial pressure (Box 8.2). The LP ventilation model needed specific boundary conditions set for respiratory rate and respiratory tidal volume (Box 8.2). The baseline boundary conditions were estimated by using the patient age, weight, and height to estimate the metabolic rate, oxygen uptake, ventilation rate (or minute ventilation), and cardiac output.[1] The resting respiratory rate was assumed to be 12 breaths per minute, and the resting heart rate was assumed to be 65 beats per minute. Metabolic demand was assumed to stay at a baseline value so that during the simulation of gas exchange, the values of venous O_2 and CO_2 were updated to maintain a constant baseline metabolic rate. The 3D ventilation of the lung was assumed to be constant. Only constant baseline values of cardiac output and minute ventilation were used in the LP model in assessing hypoxemic risk in individual APE patients.[1] The LP model calculated the maximum derangement in arterial blood O_2 and CO_2 values as the hypoxemic risk and hypercapnic risk, respectively.[1] The LP model also assessed the elevation of mean pulmonary artery pressure (mPAP), which provides a direct indication of right ventricular afterload. The increase in right ventricular afterload is what can produce acute right ventricular failure and death in APE.

RESULTS OF LUNG PHYSIOME MODEL IN PREDICTING HYPOXEMIC RISK IN APE

The LP model calculated the systemic arterial partial pressure of oxygen (PaO_2) in order to assess the presence of hypoxemia, decreased levels of oxygen in systemic arterial blood. Hypoxemia is present when the PaO_2 is less than 80 mm Hg (Box 8.3).[1]

> **BOX 8.3 ■ LP Perfusion Model Outputs for Assessment of Hypoxemic Risk**
>
> **Systemic Arterial Partial Pressure of Oxygen, PaO$_2$**
> - Hypoxemia present if PaO$_2$ is <80 mm Hg
>
> **Systemic Arterial Partial Pressure of Carbon Dioxide, PaCO$_2$**
> - Hypercapnia present if PaCO$_2$ is >54 mm Hg

The LP model calculated the partial pressure of carbon dioxide (PaCO$_2$) in order to assess the presence of systemic artery hypercapnia, elevated levels of carbon dioxide in systemic arterial blood. Hypercapnia is present when the PaCO$_2$ is greater than 54 mm Hg (Box 8.3). Eight of the 12 patients with APE in Tawhai's study were predicted to have hypoxemia, and 11 of the 12 patients with APE were predicted to have hypercapnia.[1] Each of the eight patients that the LP model predicted hypoxemia was identified clinically as having right ventricular dysfunction. The four patients the LP model predicted would not have hypoxemia did not have clinical evidence of right ventricular (RV) dysfunction. However, the calculated blood clot load had significant overlap between the patients clinically identified as having RV dysfunction and those that did not have clinical evidence of RV dysfunction. The presence of systemic arterial hypoxemia drives the cardiorespiratory system to compensate by increasing pulmonary artery systolic pressure (sPAP). The increase in sPAP increases the peak pressure the right ventricle must generate. This can produce RV dysfunction and acute RV failure.

The LP model calculation of PaO$_2$ showed a strong correlation with the measured sPAP in the 12 patients included in this study, $R^2 = 0.84057$ (Table 8.1). The clot burden load as measured by the Qanadli obstruction index (QOI) was weakly correlated with sPAP, $R^2 = 0.27219$ (Table 8.1). The LP estimate of PaO$_2$ was a much better predictor of sPAP and the risk of RV dysfunction than the QOI (Table 8.1). This illustrates the power of the LP model that combines patient-specific 3D CT lung structure information with computer modeling of lung function. The LP model predictions of both PaO$_2$ and mPAP were highly correlated to clinical measures of sPAP and the ratio of right ventricular to left ventricular volume ratios than the QOI (Table 8.1).

The LP model prediction of sPAP is better than the QOI prediction of sPAP because the LP model takes into account the 3D position of the clot in the lung. A blood clot in the lower lung that is occluding a pulmonary artery in that location will produce a greater decrease in gas exchange because the ventilation to the lower lung is greater than the ventilation in the upper lung. A blood clot in the upper lung will not decrease the gas exchange as much as in the lower lung because the ventilation in the upper lung is less than the ventilation in the lower lung. The LP model also accounts for another process that leads to decreased gas exchange with resultant hypoxemia and hypercapnia. The LP model accounts for blood flow that is diverted away from the region of the lung that has a blood clot, and this results in increased perfusion in areas of lung that produces a decrease in the ventilation to perfusion ratio (V/Q) in the regions of lung without a blood clot. This decrease in V/Q ratio will also decrease gas exchange in the lung and increase hypoxemia and hypercapnia. Patient-specific hypoxemic risk calculated by the LP model using patient-specific 3D lung CT angiogram in APE patients was a much

TABLE 8.1 ■ Results of the LP Perfusion Model in Assessing Hypoxemic Risk in Patients With Suspected APE

	sPAP (mm Hg)	RV/LV
QOI percentage	$R^2 = 0.27219$	$R^2 = 0.4279$
LP model percentage increase in mPAP	$R^2 = 0.73119$	$R^2 = 0.82182$
LP model percentage decrease in PaO$_2$	$R^2 = 0.84057$	$R^2 = 0.7562$

(Data from Tawhai MH, Clark AR, Chase JG. The lung physiome and virtual patient models: from morphometry to clinical translation. *Morphologie*. 2019;103(343):131–138, Fig. 1).

stronger predictor of right ventricular dysfunction than standard clinical metrics or clot burden scores that are also derived from a 3D lung CT angiogram.[1]

EXTENDING THE LUNG PHYSIOME MODEL APPROACH TO USING GENERIC VASCULAR ANATOMY

The use of the LP model to predict hypoxemia, hypercapnia, and increased sPAP with RV dysfunction requires a patient-specific 3D lung CT angiogram as described above in *"Results of Lung Physiome Model in Predicting Hypoxemic Risk in APE"*. The question is whether a generic vascular anatomy with realistic clot location can be used in a generic model to predict patient-specific values of mPAP and PaO$_2$.[1] Tawhai investigated the performance of a generic model in the LP model for APE.[1] One of the 12 patient models was chosen to be the generic lung model. The 3D CTPA from one of the 12 subjects was selected to provide the structural information for the model. This model was customized to each of the other 11 patients in the study by scaling the lung volume and patient-specific diameters of vessels and airways to the subsegmental level. The 3D CTPA images of the specific patient were used to identify the size and distribution of the clots in each of the 12 patients. This generic approach, using only a single rescaled 3D CTPA study, produced a generic LP model that predicted reasonable mean values of mPAP and PaO$_2$. Unfortunately, one-third of the generic LP patient models underestimated the mPAP value, and in half of the generic LP patient models the hypoxemic risk was overestimated.[1] These results highlight the added value of providing patient-specific lung structure derived from each patient's 3D CTPA images to the LP model.[1]

Summary of Important Concepts of the Lung Physiome Model

The patient-specific lung anatomy provided by the 3D CTPA provided essential lung structural information for the LP model, including 3D lung volume, airways, and pulmonary arteries and veins. A lung physiome model of pulmonary circulation that only considers the pulmonary circulation without considering the gravitationally deformed lung tissue surrounding these vessels will miss the important contribution of the preferential distribution of blood flow in the lung due to gravity.[1] A lung physiome model that only considers the pre-acinar blood vessels cannot accurately represent the recruitment of acinar capillary beds away from the acini that have under-perfused capillary beds because they are distal to blood clots occluding the upstream pulmonary artery.[1] Finally, lung physiome models that replace most of the pulmonary artery tree with "structured outflow" boundary conditions will not account for most of the mechanisms that determine pulmonary blood flow distribution in the human lung.[1]

The physiomics approach to human health and disease could play a vital role in constructing increasingly sophisticated and more capable predictive models of human health and disease. The use of a lung physiome model, such as the LP model, can be envisioned to work inside a comprehensive AI framework in routine clinical imaging along with the other reactive and limited-memory AI methods that have been described in Chapters 4, 5, 6, and 7. Chapter 9 will discuss the current lung CT AI models that are available for routine clinical use.

References

1. Tawhai MH, Clark AR, Chase JG. The lung physiome and virtual patient models: from morphometry to clinical translation. *Morphologie*. 2019;103(343):131–138.
2. Crampin EJ, Halstead M, Hunter P, Nielsen P, Noble D, Smith N, et al. Computational physiology and the Physiome Project. *Exp Physiol*. 2004;89(1):1–26.
3. Wikipedia, The Free Encyclopedia. Physiome. Updated December 13, 2020. Accessed June 29, 2022. Available at: https://en.wikipedia.org/wiki/Physiome.
4. Tawhai M, Clark A, Donovan G, Burrowes K. Computational modeling of airway and pulmonary vascular structure and function: development of a "lung physiome". *Crit Rev Biomed Eng*. 2011;39(4):319–336.
5. Clark AR, Milne D, Wilsher M, Burrowes KS, Bajaj M, Tawhai MH. Lack of functional information explains the poor performance of 'clot load scores' at predicting outcome in acute pulmonary embolism. *Respir Physiol Neurobiol*. 2014;190:1–13.
6. Clark AR, Tawhai MH, Hoffman EA, Burrowes KS. The interdependent contributions of gravitational and structural features to perfusion distribution in a multiscale model of the pulmonary circulation. *J Appl Physiol (1985)*. 2011;110(4):943–955.
7. Kang W, Clark AR, Tawhai MH. Gravity outweighs the contribution of structure to passive ventilation-perfusion matching in the supine adult human lung. *J Appl Physiol (1985)*. 2018;124(1):23–33.
8. Swan AJ, Clark AR, Tawhai MH. A computational model of the topographic distribution of ventilation in healthy human lungs. *J Theor Biol*. 2012;300:222–231.
9. Burrowes KS, Clark AR, Marcinkowski A, Wilsher ML, Milne DG, Tawhai MH. Pulmonary embolism: predicting disease severity. *Philos Trans A Math Phys Eng Sci*. 2011;369(1954):4255–4277.
10. Chase JG, Preiser JC, Dickson JL, Pironet A, Chiew YS, Pretty CG, et al. Next-generation, personalised, model-based critical care medicine: a state-of-the-art review of in silico virtual patient models, methods, and cohorts, and how to validation them. *Biomed Eng Online*. 2018;17(1):24.
11. Clark AR, Burrowes KS, Tawhai MH. Contribution of serial and parallel microperfusion to spatial variability in pulmonary inter- and intra-acinar blood flow. *J Appl Physiol (1985)*. 2010;108(5):1116–1126.
12. Albrecht MH, Bickford MW, Nance Jr. JW, Zhang L, De Cecco CN, Wichmann JL, et al. State-of-the-art pulmonary CT angiography for acute pulmonary embolism. *Am J Roentgenol*. 2017;208(3):495–504.

Adoption of Lung CT AI Into Clinical Medicine

Introduction

The successes in the 2000s and 2010s in developing reactive machine AI and limited-memory AI methods to detect and assess the present and severity of x-ray chest CT imaging findings associated with COVID-19 pneumonia, COPD, ILD, and lung cancer have spurred the development of multiple quantitative CT (QCT) lung AI companies, such as VIDA, that offer point-of-care lung CT AI products to assess lung diseases. VIDA's specialized FDA-approved lung CT AI program, VIDA Insights v3.0, can be run independently or inside a larger medical imaging AI ecosystem. It is now possible for every chest CT scan to be analyzed in near real time for QCT AI metrics of COVID-19 pneumonia, COPD, ILD, and lung nodules. The lung CT AI information is automatically generated and inserted in imaging physicians' reports and have an immediate impact on the detection and assessment of the severity of diffuse lung disease and lung cancer. It has been a long journey from the mid-1970s to the early 2020s, but QCT AI of lung disease for the clinical care and treatment of COPD and ILD is now coming of age.

Healthcare Imaging IT

Imaging technology in modern healthcare systems relies on an ecosystem of AI agents to deliver high-quality medical care to patients. The AI agents covered in this chapter include the electronic medical record, radiology information system, picture archiving and communication, voice recognition and reporting, and disease-specific quantitative lung CT AI agents.

Electronic Medical Record (EMR)

The EMR is an AI program that stores, transmits, and displays critical medical information for a patient seen within a healthcare organization (e.g., clinic, hospital, web).[1] The EMR is used by medical personnel to care for patients. The EMR is interfaced with other AI programs that perform more specialized AI functions, such as medical imaging. The medical imaging AI programs include picture archiving and communication (PACS) software programs, radiology information system (RIS) software programs, and voice recognition and reporting (VR) software programs. The PACS, RIS, and VR programs all work together to enable imaging physicians to create imaging reports on the medical imaging studies contained in the PACS and then have these same imaging reports sent to the EMR where they can be viewed by the ordering physician and the other healthcare workers and the patient.

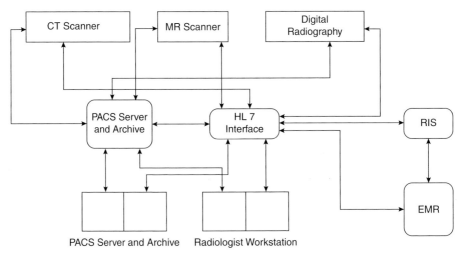

Fig. 9.1 Computer network relationships between different medical informatics technologies including the CT scanner, Radiologist Workstation, PACS Server/Archive, HL Interface, and RIS.

PICTURE ARCHIVING AND COMMUNICATION SYSTEM (PACS)

The PACS is the core technology that is responsible for storing, transmitting, and displaying medical images within healthcare systems. The major PACS components include hardware, software, and local area networks (Fig. 9.1). The hardware consists of computer servers to store and transmit medical imaging studies, computer workstations where the medical images are interpreted by imaging physicians, and local area networks that connect the medical imaging devices (e.g., x-ray CT scanners) to the computer servers that store the medical imaging data.[1] The PACS software components include the software that controls the storage and transmission of medical images, software to display and interact with the medical images, and software that exchanges information with the RIS and EMR.

The data format for medical images has been standardized using what is called the Digital Imaging and Communications in Medicine (DICOM) standard. DICOM provides standard protocols for exchanging and storing medical image data including both image data and text associated with the image data. Manufacturers of PACS software have adopted the DICOM standard. The Medical and Imaging Technical Alliance (MITA) division of the National Electrical Manufacturers Association (NEMA) manages a structured document describing the DICOM standard. The DICOM Standard's document currently includes 20 Parts, Parts 1–8, Parts 10–12, and Parts 14–22.[1] Each of the DICOM Standard Parts address specific subject areas, for example Part 10 addresses "Media Storage and File Format for Media Interchange".[1,2] The International Organization for Standardization has recognized DICOM as the ISO 10252 standard.[2]

The development of web-based PACS software has driven the need to develop an application programming interface (API) for handling DICOM-compliant medical imaging data on the worldwide web. DICOMweb has been developed to provide an

API to support DICOM standards for web applications similar to what DICOM standards have done for PACS systems. The DICOMweb API provides software programming standards for web-based medical imaging applications for sending, retrieving, and querying images and image-related information.[1]

Current PACS systems provide for "hanging protocols" to be assigned to each type of imaging study. Hanging protocols are implemented within the DICOM standard.[1,2] The term "hanging" comes from the historic method of hanging hardcopy film on a viewer for the imaging physician to visually interpret and report the findings of a given imaging study. The PACS hanging protocols provide powerful tools to organize the display of the different imaging studies, such as chest CT scans. The hanging protocols are not specific to a patient but are specific to the type of imaging study performed. The chest CT hanging protocol can include multiple parameters including anatomic laterality (right versus left), the anatomic plane that is displayed (e.g., axial, coronal, sagittal), reconstruction method (FBP versus IR), reconstruction kernel, slice thickness, slice interval, window width (WW), window level (WL), location on the displays of the current chest CT images, and historic chest CT's if they exist.[1] A lung CT AI program that produces additional DICOM outputs needs to be able to integrate into the hanging protocol of the different PACS vendor systems. This is usually done by generating a new CT series that can be handled by the PACS like any other CT imaging series.

RADIOLOGY INFORMATION SOFTWARE (RIS)

The RIS is a medical information AI agent that communicates through the medical imaging LAN network with the EHR to send and receive patient-specific medical imaging study information. The RIS has recently been incorporated into the EMR rather than continue to be a stand-alone software program. The RIS typically has imaging modality and subspecialty-specific worklists that inform the imaging physician and the imaging technologist as to which patients need a specific imaging study (e.g., chest CT) and why the specific imaging study was ordered. The RIS has access to patient-specific information stored in the EHR to inform the imaging physician as to why the medical imaging examination was ordered (e.g., patient chief complaint and symptoms), and to receive the structured reporting documents generated by the imaging physician, usually using VR reporting software. The RIS software sends the report on the medical imaging study back to the EMR to update the patient's electronic medical record.

The communication standards between the EMR, RIS, and PACS are implemented using the HL7 standard.[1,3] Health Level Seven International (HL7) was founded in 1987. HL7 is a non-profit organization that develops ANSI-accredited framework and standards for the exchange, integration, and sharing of electronic health information. The HL7 standard provides a mechanism for the electronic exchange of alphanumeric medical information (e.g., text and numbers) between the different software programs that are running on a medical informatics local area network (LAN), including the EMR, RIS, PACS, and other medical informatics programs in the healthcare IT environment, such as the Laboratory Information System (LIS).[1]

MEDICAL IMAGING REPORTING AND VOICE RECOGNITION SOFTWARE (VR)

Every medical imaging study needs to be visually assessed and an accurate and concise report generated for the imaging study. Voice recognition (VR) software has been used in reporting medical imaging studies over the past couple of decades. The currently available versions of the FDA-approved VR reporting software are quite capable and in use by most imaging physicians. The most popular VR reporting software for imaging studies including CT is Nuance's AI-driven PowerScribe 360 and PowerScribe One.

Clinical Lung CT AI Software

The development of clinical lung CT AI software to detect and assess lung disease must be able to fit into the larger medical imaging IT environment previously described. The goal of clinical lung CT AI software should be to accurately assess chest CT studies for quantitative metrics of lung disease while integrating smoothly into the clinical imaging workflow. This means that the lung CT AI software needs to access chest CT imaging data either directly from the x-ray CT scanner or the PACS. The lung CT AI software needs to run quickly in the background so that the results are available when the chest CT study is interpreted by the imaging physician. The outputs from the lung CT AI software need to be DICOM compliant for results that are stored in the PACS with the chest CT study that has been analyzed. The HL7-compliant alpha-numeric outputs from the lung CT AI program, such as LAA_{-950} for the assessment of emphysema, should be able to flow into the VR reports along with other structured text reporting fields.

VIDA INSIGHTS–CLINICAL LUNG CT AI SOFTWARE

As of December 2021, VIDA Insights has two modules: Density/tMPR and Texture/Subpleural View.[4] VIDA lung CT AI software is rapidly evolving, and the latest information on VIDA lung CT AI can be accessed on the web.[4] VIDA Insights can be integrated with the CT scanner PACS (Fig. 9.2).

VIDA Insights assesses each of the imaging series obtained for the chest CT study and finds the study with the best technique for assessing the lungs. This includes looking for a contiguous data acquisition with a slice thickness of 1.5 mm or less and FBP reconstruction with a neutral kernel (see Chapter 3). Then, the selected series is automatically analyzed by a deep learning AI software program to see if there are motion artifacts within the lungs. VIDA Insights will use the results of these quality control steps to inform the imaging physician as to the acceptability of the chest CT in question. If there are severe quality issues, then the chest CT will not be analyzed.

VIDA Insights automatically segments the lungs and airways from the rest of the thoracic anatomy using a deep learning AI software program. The lung segmentation is robust and includes segmenting the individual lungs and lobes. The challenge of separating the lungs from the mediastinal and chest wall structures automatically and accurately is substantial, since a peripheral area of consolidation from COVID-19 pneumonia that abuts the pleura or diaphragm has similar tissue densities. Robust lung CT

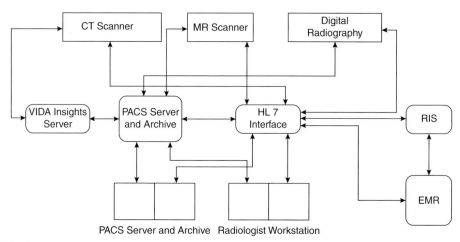

Fig. 9.2 The integration of VIDA Insights server that can be done with the CT scanner(s) and the PACS Server/Archive.

image segmentation is an ongoing research-and-development process pursued through public and industry-funded research.

The design of VIDA Insights was modeled after the method a thoracic radiologist applies to the visual interpretation of the lung findings on a chest CT study. This includes finding the best CT image series to assess the lungs and checking that the chest CT scan was done at the correct lung volume, with the correct chest CT scan protocol, and ensuring there are no motion artifacts that will adversely affect the visual interpretation of the lung CT images. Then, the lungs are assessed for evidence of increased, normal, or decreased lung volumes. Increased lung volumes are associated with obstructive airway diseases, such as COPD and asthma. Decreased lung volumes are associated with restrictive lung diseases, such as ILD. Normal or near-normal lung volumes are associated with acute lung disease, such as COVID-19 pneumonia. Next, the lung CT images are assessed for areas of decreased density due to emphysema, or increased density due to pneumonia or pulmonary fibrosis. Then, the lung CT images are assessed for characteristic texture patterns of diseased lung tissue: ground-glass/reticular opacities, consolidation, and honeycombing.

VIDA Insights Density/tMPR Reactive Machine AI Tool for Assessing Volumes, LAA, and HAA

Chapter 5 discussed the COPDGene study use of four novel criteria to diagnose COPD and to assess the impact of these criteria on COPD progression and mortality: "Exposure, Symptoms, CT Structural Abnormality, Spirometry".[5] Exposure was defined as having a 10-pack-year or greater smoking history[5] Symptoms were defined as self-reporting a modified Medical Council (mMRC) dyspnea score of 2 or greater and/or chronic bronchitis (self-reported chronic cough and phlegm).[5] CT structural abnormality was defined as having one or more of the following: LAA_{-950} equal to 5% or greater on a TLC chest CT scan (QCT structural measure of emphysema), $LAA_{-856} \geq 15\%$ on expiratory CT scan (QCT functional measure of air trapping), Pi10 equal to 2.5 mm or

Density

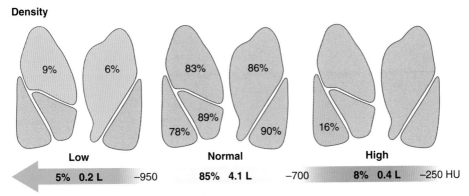

Fig. 9.3 VIDA Insights Density/tMPR modules' graphical output for the lung and lobe volumes in a patient with upper lobe emphysema and right lower lobe pulmonary fibrosis, ground-glass, reticulations, and traction bronchiectasis (see Figs. 9.6 and 9.7). The LAA$_{-950}$ metric to assess emphysema is displayed on the left as Low: 5% by volume with lobes >5% highlighted in yellow. The HAA$_{-700 \text{ to } -250}$ metric is displayed on the right as High: 8% by volume with lobes >10% highlighted in blue, to assess pneumonia and interstitial lung abnormalities. The amount of normal lung is displayed in the middle graphic as Normal: 85% by volume.

	Total	Right	Left	RUL	RML	RLL	LUL	LLL
Volume (L)	4.8	2.3	2.5	1.1	0.5	0.8	1.3	1.2
Low density (%)	5	5	4	9	3	2	6	2
High density (%)	8	10	7	7	7	16	6	7
Normal density (%)	85	82	88	83	89	78	86	90

Fig. 9.4 VIDA Insights Density/tMPR modules tabular output for the lung and lobe volumes for the same patient as in Fig. 9.3. Whole lung, individual lung, and lobe volumes, LAA$_{-950}$, HAA$_{-700 \text{ to } -250}$ are shown in the table.

greater (QCT structural measure of airway wall thickening).[5] The results of this study provide guidance and value to assessing the LAA$_{-950}$ to detect and assess emphysema in a clinical lung CT AI program.

VIDA Insights Density/tMPR assessment uses a reactive machine AI approach to analyze the lung voxel histogram curve obtained from each lung and lobe from the segmented lung CT images. The volume of each lung and lobe can be calculated by knowing the volume of each lung CT voxel and the number of lung CT voxels in each lung and lobe. The lung and lobe volumes are calculated by multiplying the volume of each voxel by the number of voxels in each lobe and lung, and the volume is expressed in liters for each lung and lobe.

VIDA Insights Density/tMPR then analyzes the lung CT voxel histogram curve to calculate the number of voxels <−950 HU or the LAA$_{-950}$ discussed in Chapter 5. The LAA$_{-950}$ is a QCT metric of emphysema and when the LAA$_{-950}$ is 5% or greater, the affected lung or lobe is highlighted in yellow (Figs. 9.3 and 9.4). As the percentage of LAA$_{-950}$ increases above 5%, the color deepens in the affected lung and lobe.

Chapter 5 also discussed that Podolanczuk et al. in 2016 reported results using a QCT lung metric referred to as *high attenuating areas* (HAA) to assess preclinical evidence of interstitial lung abnormalities in middle-aged and older adult community-dwelling population.[6] The HAA in this study was defined as the amount of lung that is between −600 HU and −250 HU. The HAA represents increases in lung densities as opposed to the LAA that reports decreases in lung density. Podolanczuk concluded that the HAA QCT metric was a valid QCT phenotype of subclinical lung injury and lung inflammation and that it may be a precursor to subclinical interstitial lung disease (ILD). HAA can be used to assess early as well as more advanced cases of ILD. The results of this study provide guidance and value to assessing the HAA to detect and assess ILD in a clinical lung CT AI program.

Chapter 5 also discussed how Colombi et al. reported in 2020 that assessing the amount of well-aerated lung using visual lung CT or lung CT AI in patients with confirmed COVID-19 viral pneumonia was better predictor of ICU admission or death compared to using nonimaging clinical parameters.[7] The lung CT AI method first segmented the normal lungs from the rest of the thoracic anatomy. Then, the percent of the lung CT voxels between −950 HU and −700 HU were used to calculate the percentage of normally aerated lung, %S-WAL. The absolute volume of well-aerated lung was also calculated. If the amount of well-aerated lung, %S-WAL, was <71%, the odds that the patient would be in the ICU/Death group increased by 3.7. If the volume of well-aerated lung, VOL-WAL, was <2.9 liters, the odds that the patient would be in the ICU/Death group increased by 2.6.[7]

The work of Podolanczuk and Colombi, along with internal research, has led VIDA to calculate a value of HAA between −700 HU and −250 HU on noncontrast TLC CT scans to assess HAA produced by COVID-19 acute viral pneumonia, ILD, and other forms of lung disease that increase lung density.

VIDA Insights Density/tMPR analyzes the lung CT voxel histogram curve to calculate $HAA_{-700 \text{ to } -250}$, which is the number of voxels with a value in HU between −700 HU and −250 HU (Figs. 9.3 and 9.4). When the $HAA_{-700 \text{ to } -250}$ is ≥10%, the lobe or lung is highlighted in blue. As the percentage $HAA_{-700 \text{ to } -250}$ increases above 10% in the affected lung or lobe, the color deepens (Fig. 9.3).

VIDA Discovery Limited-Memory AI Texture Tool

In Chapter 7 we discussed how Humphries et al. in 2017 described a novel unsupervised limited AI agent that could identify fibrotic lung regions, for example, combinations of reticular opacities (RO), honeycombing (HO), and traction bronchiectasis (TB), in patients with interstitial lung disease from idiopathic pulmonary fibrosis (IPF).[8] There were significant correlations in this study between baseline data-driven textural analysis (DTA) fibrotic score, mean lung density, skewness, kurtosis and visual assessment of fibrosis, and baseline values of FVC and DLCO.[8] The QCT metrics correlated better with baseline FVC and DLCO than the visual scoring method. There were significant correlations in the change of the DTA score (lung fibrosis) mean lung density, skewness, kurtosis and visual assessment of fibrosis, and the change in FVC in the 72 IPF subjects with baseline and follow-up chest CT scans, and measures of FVC and DLCO. The quantitative measures, again, outperformed the visual scores. The change in the DTA score, mean lung density, skewness, and visual score significantly correlated with the

Texture

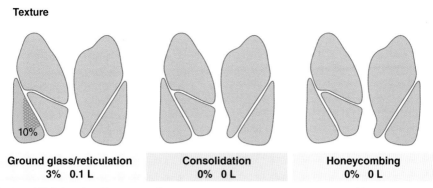

Ground glass/reticulation	Consolidation	Honeycombing
3% 0.1 L	0% 0 L	0% 0 L

Fig. 9.5 VIDA Insights Texture module output for the same patient shown in Figs. 9.3 and 9.4. The VIDA Insights Texture module identified ground-glass and/or reticulations in 10% by volume of the right lower lobe, blue color. The ground-glass and/or reticulations in the right lower lobe was equal to 3% per 0.1 liter of the total lung volume. VIDA Insights Texture module did not identify any consolidation or honeycombing in the lungs.

change in DLCO. The change in DTA score and visual score outperformed the change in mean lung density and skewness in assessing the change in DLCO from baseline to follow-up.[8] The results of Humphries's study provide guidance and value in assessing texture patterns in patients with IPF and other ILDs.

When VIDA Insights Density/tMPR module assesses a chest CT scan and there are >10% HAA abnormalities present, the VIDA Insights Texture/Subpleural View module can be run to assess what texture patterns are present in the areas of lung with HAA abnormalities. The Texture/Subpleural View tool evaluates the amount by volume of lung affected with ground-glass and/or reticulations, consolidation, and honeycombing. The texture tool is a limited-memory AI agent that uses supervised deep machine learning methods to identify the presence and assess the extent of ground-glass/reticulations, consolidation, and honeycombing within the areas of HAA (Fig. 9.5).

Enhanced Visualization of Airways and Subpleural Lung Tissue

VIDA Insights, as of December 2021, has two modules, Density/tMPR and Texture/Subpleural View, which can automatically provide quantitative metrics of diffuse lung disease and also enhanced visualizations of the airways and subpleural lung tissue. The Density/tMPR module provides an enhanced visual assessment of the larger central airways, generations 1–4, and the adjacent lung tissue (Fig. 9.6). This enhanced visualization of the airways provides a more efficient method of detecting mucus plugs, bronchiectasis, airway wall thickening, and endobronchial tumors. The Texture/Subpleural View provides an enhanced visual assessment of the subpleural lung tissue (Fig. 9.7). The enhanced visualization of the subpleural space makes it possible to view and rapidly assess the entire subpleural space for the presence of subpleural honeycombing in patients with ILD.

VIDA Lung Nodule Tool

VIDA is developing an automatic lung nodule detection and assessment tool to increase the efficiency of imaging physicians to detect lung nodules, and also to provide AI tools to

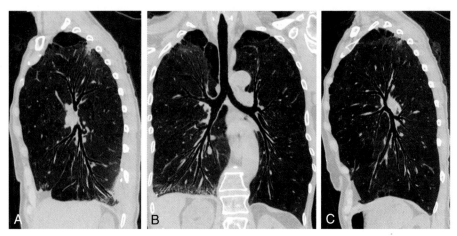

Fig. 9.6   These three airway tMPR images are from the same patient shown in Figs. 9.3, 9.4, and 9.5. **(A)** Right sagittal tMPR image showing the airways in the right lung. **(B)** Coronal tMPR shows the airways of both lungs. **(C)** Left sagittal tMPR image showing the airways of the left lung. There are low-density areas of emphysema in both upper lungs and there are areas of ground-glass and reticulations with traction bronchiectasis in the right lower lung.

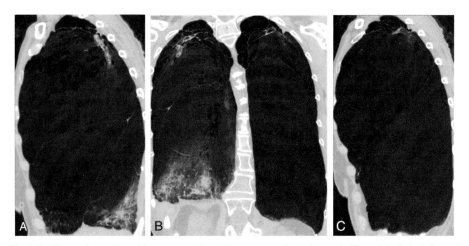

Fig. 9.7   These three pleural images are from the same patient shown in Figs. 9.3, 9.4, 9.5, and 9.6. The subpleural images optimally assess the entire subpleural lung tissue, 1 mm from the visceral pleural surface. **(A)** Lateral subpleural view of the right lung. **(B)** Posterior subpleural view of both lungs. **(C)** Lateral subpleural view of the left lung. These subpleural views show upper lobe predominant decreased density in the areas of subpleural emphysema in both lungs. There are also areas of increased density in the right lower lobe due to ground-glass and reticular opacities due to subpleural pulmonary fibrosis.

assess the risk of cancer in the detected lung nodules. We discussed in Chapter 4 the value of AI methods to assess lung nodule volumes and the risk of malignancies. We also indicated the need to automatically detect the lung nodules and segment them from the rest of the lung tissue automatically. These goals are driving the design of VIDA's lung nodule tool.

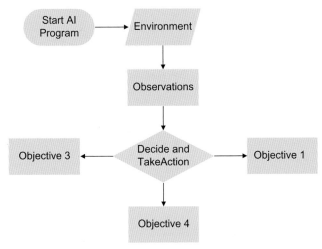

Fig. 9.8   Relationships of the four principal components of an AI agent.

VIDA Discovery Lung Ventilation Tool

VIDA has developed software tools to assess air trapping when both inspiratory and expiratory CT scans have been obtained (see Chapter 6). There is a lot of interest in a clinical lung CT AI tool to assess air trapping on expiratory CT scans. VIDA can provide measures of air trapping through the VIDA Discovery software product.[4] VIDA Discovery has the ability to transfer anonymized CT image data over the internet in an efficient and largely automated process to VIDA Research Imaging Analysts. These analysts grow the airway tree and label the airways. They verify image segmentation and image registration so that DPM methods can be used to provide variable threshold voxel-based measurements of small airway disease, associated air trapping, and emphysema (see Chapter 6). VIDA's DPM method (see Chapter 6) uses both TLC and FRC/RV chest CT scans to perform nonrigid registration of these images so that normal lung tissue, air trapping without emphysema, air trapping with emphysema, and emphysema without air trapping can be assessed at the voxel level.

Responsible AI

Stuart Russell in his book *Human Compatible* describes the key concept in modern artificial intelligence (AI) as being the concept of an intelligent agent (see Chapter 1).[9] The intelligent agent exists in the software program(s) running on a computer(s). How the AI agent is built depends on the objective(s) we want to achieve or the problem we want to solve. The functioning AI agent then depends on four important things: environment, observations, actions, and objective(s) (Fig. 9.8).[9] The environment is the physical and electronic space that the AI agent can access. The central concept of modern AI is that of an intelligent agent that runs in an environment that the AI agent can observe and from these observations take action(s) to achieve an objective(s).[9]

Responsible AI is concerned with how humans ensure that humans will remain in control of AI and that the objective(s) of AI software agents align well with accepted

BOX 9.1 ■ **Three Principles of Responsible AI**

1. Purely altruistic AI machine
2. Humble AI machine
3. AI machine learns how to predict human preferences

ethical standards and moral values of human societies. Russell describes three principles for designing a beneficial AI machine. The first principle is a purely altruistic machine. The second principle is a humble machine. The third principle is a machine that learns to predict human preferences (Box 9.1).[9] Russell goes on to describe in his book that it is possible to design AI agents that incorporate these three principles and that the AI agents can be designed to be provably beneficial and safe.[9] The levels of AI that we have considered in this book are the two most basic levels: reactive machine and limited-memory. The more advanced levels of AI, Theory of Mind AI and Self-Aware AI—are not currently implemented in medical imaging, to the best of my knowledge, nor have they been implemented in other areas. However, even the reactive machine and limited-memory AI agents need to be designed with care in medical imaging.

I think it is important to consider how best to implement responsible AI in medical imaging. We have seen significant advances in lung CT AI from the first digital CT images of the lung in 1975 to the remarkable limited-memory AI agents we described in Chapter 7 that can extract image features that a human cannot, and do it in a precise and quantitative manner. It is reasonable to assume that lung CT AI will continue to advance at a rapid pace. The idea that a lung CT AI agent can be altruistic or unselfish is embodied in the idea that any AI analysis of the lung CT images will be subject to review in a meaningful way by the human imaging physician. This can be in the form of labeling lung CT images with different colors to represent different objectives for example, yellow for LAA and blue for HAA. The lung CT AI agent can be humble in agreeing to let the human imaging physician reject the results of the lung CT AI agent. Currently, to learn the preferences of the human imaging physician, the lung CT AI agent designers, humans, need to get meaningful feedback on the user interface that the lung CT AI agent uses to present results. This is a dynamic process that needs to continue for the entire time the lung CT AI agent is used. The actual metrics that the lung CT AI agent produces to detect and assess underlying disease need to be scientifically sound and transparent. This is easier to achieve when reactive machine-type AI agents are used, such as assessing decreases in lung density from emphysema by assessing the number of voxels <-950 HU. It is more difficult when a deep machine learning strategy is used where the hidden layers in a convolutional neural net may be hard to assess for a human imaging physician. I think here caution is in order. One safe approach is to have the deep learning AI agent analyze patterns that have already been labeled as abnormal by a simpler reactive machine AI strategy and to make sure that the deep learning AI outputs can be projected back onto the lung CT images to see if, for example, the deep learning AI assessment of honeycombing is mapped to the lung CT images so they can be reviewed easily by the human imaging physician.

It is the responsibility of all stakeholders in the lung CT AI community to design and implement responsible AI agents. Following Stuart Russell's three principles of responsible AI in the development of lung CT AI agents will help ensure that lung CT AI agents serve the needs of human health now and in the future.

References

1. Bushberg JT, Seibert JA, Leidholdt Jr EM, Boone JM. *Medical Imaging Informatics. The Essential Physics of Medical Imaging*. 4th ed. Mexico City, Mexico: Wolters Kluwer; 2021:109–181.
2. DICOM. Current Edition. Accessed June 30, 2022. Available at: https://www.dicomstandard.org/current.
3. HL7. HL7 International Website 2021. Accessed April 29, 2022. Available at: http://www.hl7.org.
4. VIDA. VIDA Website 2021. Accessed April 29, 2022. Available at: https://vidalung.ai.
5. Lowe KE, Regan EA, Anzueto A, Austin E, Austin JHM, Beaty TH, et al. COPDGene® 2019. Redefining the diagnosis of chronic obstructive pulmonary disease. *Chronic Obstr Pulm Dis*. 2019;6(5):384–399.
6. Podolanczuk AJ, Oelsner EC, Barr RG, Hoffman EA, Armstrong HF, Austin JH, et al. High attenuation areas on chest computed tomography in community-dwelling adults: the MESA study. *Eur Respir J*. 2016;48(5):1442–1452.
7. Colombi D, Bodini FC, Petrini M, Maffi G, Morelli N, Milanese G, et al. Well-aerated lung on admitting chest CT to predict adverse outcome in COVID-19 pneumonia. *Radiology*. 2020;296(2):E86–E96.
8. Humphries SM, Yagihashi K, Huckleberry J, Rho BH, Schroeder JD, Strand M, et al. Idiopathic pulmonary fibrosis: data-driven textural analysis of extent of fibrosis at baseline and 15-month follow-up. *Radiology*. 2017;285(1):270–278.
9. Russell S. *Human Compatible: Artificial Intelligence and the Problem of Control*. New York, NY: Viking Press; 2019:1–256.

Note: Page numbers followed by *f*, *t*, and *b* indicate figures, tables, and boxes, respectively.